Dark

Cures

Have Doctors Lost Their Ethics?

by Paul deParrie

Huntington House Publishers

Huntington House Publishers
P.O. Box 53788
Lafayette, Louisiana 70505

Library of Congress Card Catalog Number
95-77223
ISBN 1-56384-099-5

Unless otherwise indicated,
all Scripture quotations are taken from the
King James Version of the Bible.

Printed in the U.S.A.

114105

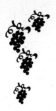

Dedication

To the souls who remain anonymous, who hazard their lives for the sake of life: You will hear, "Well done, thou good and faithful servant" from the most important Voice. Then you will be anonymous no longer.

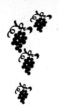

Contents

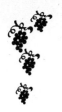

Acknowledgments

I would like to express my gratitude to my sponsoring editor at Huntington House Publishers, who worked hard to get this work published. I am also very grateful to my two most critical editors, my wife, Bonnie, and my friend and co-worker, Cathy Ramey, without whom this manuscript would have been far less readable. I am also indebted to Dr. Hilton Terrell, editor for the *Journal of Biblical Medical Ethics*, and Dr. Don Russell, who formerly was involved in tissue transplants, who both checked for possible medical inaccuracies and challenged some of my conclusions.

"Iron sharpeneth iron; so a man sharpeneth the countenance of his friend" (Prov. 27:17).

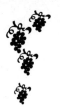

Introduction

Medicine is a wonderful thing. God has blessed man with the ability to search out many of the mysteries of the universe, including the internal universe of the human body. In doing so, we have been able to uncover the sources of many diseases and conditions which plague us as fallen man. We have been able to alleviate suffering, correct disabilities, and generally make life longer and more pleasant for a large portion of humanity. Some diseases have been nearly banished from the face of the earth. Others have been held at bay. The sick have found healing, the lame have walked, and the blind have regained sight—all in a limited sense, but marvelous, nonetheless. For all this, we praise God.

All this benevolence has root in a philosophy that values human life regardless of age, stage, or condition. But, the same kindly face of medicine, the healer, can be the face of a cruel tyrant if his motives deviate from a standard of value that guards human life. Medicine, lacking a life-affirming basis, becomes terrorism. This has been proven historically, Nazi Germany and Soviet Russia being the most recent examples.

Today, medicine in America has adopted a new ethic, an ethic of pragmatism—an ethic of death. Death has not only become a preferred "cure" for certain kinds of patients, but the deaths of these patients are often made into cures for others.

The ethical change has been slow but deliberate. Thanaphiles (Greek: death lovers), as I call them, have made great inroads—much of it without a peep from the Church. They have cloaked their activities in smooth and flattering words. They have talked of the complexity of the issues and hidden their motives behind nearly incomprehensible technology, and the public has simply swallowed the change from medical protection of life to medical taking of life.

In 1986, the first time I sat down to write on the subject of modern medical ethics and the dangers that it posed, I and my coauthor, Mary Pride, had previously been continually shocked and amazed at how far down the slippery slope Western medicine had slid. It was this that we sought to share in our book, *Unholy Sacrifices of the New Age*.

In that book, we explored some of what was brewing in the witches' cauldron of modern medicine. Some, unaware of what was happening, thought we were being sensationalistic. Yet, time has proven that our claims were true and that we even woefully underreported the inroads that ungodly thinking had made on the medical field—even among Christian doctors!

In some sense, *Unholy Sacrifices* was ahead of its time. Medical issues have become a much more prominent topic of general conversation than they were just a few short years ago. The proposals for nationalized health care, debates over funding of fetal experiments, the use of aborted babies' bodies for cures, and other issues have invaded the public arena. Questions about assisted suicide, living wills, and rationing health care have confronted us all.

If you or anyone you know will ever reach sixty years of age, become seriously ill, or sustain major physical injuries, you will someday have to make decisions—life and death decisions—regarding medical treatment. But, where do you start? Who do you believe? Aren't these issues just "too complex" for the average individual to sort out? Don't we need some sort of specialist—a medical ethicist—to clarify these issues?

I suppose that all depends on whether or not you believe that God has equipped His saints—each one—with the wherewithal to render a solid moral decision on such things.

And, a moral decision it is. All life and death decisions are inherently moral decisions. And, who better to make moral decisions than God's people? Actually, the technology may be complex, but the moral issues are not. Nor is this insurgence of pagan medical ethics a concern for Christians alone. Those who are not Christians are dying as readily as believers. It behooves them as well to be prepared to meet the challenges of making medical decisions in an increasingly dangerous medical arena.

Whether anyone realizes it or not, medicine has changed. The once-compassionate practice of medicine concerned itself solely with the treatment of the patient. Now, medicine is merely another instrument of social engineering. Because of this, medicine poses dangers for both the bodies and souls of men. And, because it has a different world view than it used to have, pagan medicine will inexorably lead us away from the principles of the Word of God. "All who hate Me, love death," Scripture tells us in Proverbs 8:36. And, it would seem that the medical ethicists in our day have chosen to love death.

This means that through a fascination with, if not love of death, they display their hatred of God. That seems to be their solution to so many problems. I believe that God has given His saints all things that pertain to life and godliness (2 Pet. 1:3). His Word and His Spirit can help you look through all the seeming complexities and make a wise decision.

To do that, however, you must cut through all the phony trappings and confusing language that have been placed around medical decisions. We must understand the basis for today's medical "ethics" and know what the Scriptures say should be the basis for true ethics.

In other words, we must know the most elemental principles of Scripture and how they apply to medical treatment. We must also be able to clear away the cobwebs and the clouds that divert us and understand what the real medical issues are. We must see how and why the field of medicine has changed and where it is leading us. Only then will we be fully prepared to resist its blandishments—its promises of health and utopia.

I pray this book will set you on that road.

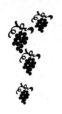

Chapter One

New Medicine for Old

1500 B.C.
Someplace on the Peloponnesian Peninsula

The shaman murmured over a bowlful of herbs as the slender old man approached his abode. The medicine man danced and shook dust and smoldering smoke over the concoction. The usually long strides of the old man were foreshortened by an apparent illness. He was here for the medicine man's cure. He slipped the payment into the offering bowl and waited for the shaman to finish the chant. "Here you are," the shaman finally said, delivering the old man a small leather bag. "This should put an end to what ails you."

Yes, the shaman was fully aware of what was good for the old man's ailment. He was fully aware that the chanting and dancing were useful only for appearance and for the aid of those superstitious among the people. The shaman was also fully cognizant that none of the herbs would help the old man. Into the potion, he had added dried nightshade. By morning, the old man's ailment would truly bother him no more! He would be dead.

Before the sun had risen that morning, one of the old man's neighbors, a secret enemy, had paid twice the amount the old man had given to insure the death of the old man for the possibility that he, the neighbor, might seize upon the land left with a mere woman and no son to guard it. No one would know of the shaman's deed. And, no matter how much some might suspect, no successful accusation could be brought against a man of his stature. Besides, the gods were with him.

The old man? Well, he and his old wife had been in poor health, always sick. They were too frail even to work their land. It was just as well. The neighbor would put the land to more profitable use.

Medicine has come a long way from the days when the local healer was really a healer/poisoner—or has it? It is possible that the most dangerous place you can be is in a hospital.

In the ancient world, those who cured the ill also mixed deadly brews. Their knowledge of herbs and minerals was quite extensive. They knew the effects of these things on the human body: whether to palliate, to heal, to make drowsy, to intoxicate, or to kill. Depending on the culture and the age, religious connotations were either omnipresent or entirely absent, but the job remained the same.

These men and women were greatly admired and feared in every society. In the Western world, however, in approximately the fourth century B.C., a man named Hippocrates began a new school of thought among his profession. He determined to completely separate the function of healing from the function of poisoning. No member of his school would have any contact with the dark side of the arts that the other schools practiced. To this end, he established an oath for his students swearing by the gods to eschew the practices of abortion, euthanasia, and any other forms of killing. There were other moral constraints they swore to as well, but those against killing were, for their time and place, the most startling.

More than just the oath, Hippocrates began treating illness rationally as opposed to imagining all sickness to be the work of gods or demons. Completely different from the going methods, Hippocrates' practices included taking extensive patient histories and using scientific investigation to search for the causes and cures of disease.

While the details of Hippocrates and his oath are lost in history, their impact remains. At the time, there were numerous schools of thought on healing, but all had accepted the common practices of varied forms of killing. Hippocrates' philosophy seemed incredible. In fact, it may have been heavily informed by his ancestry. While he was an obvious polytheist, Hippocrates was the descendant of Jewish exiles after the release from Babylon. It is possible that his odd ideas were remnants of what his family had brought with them in the Diaspora.[1]

The philosophy of healing that Hippocrates taught was just one of many competing philosophies over the centuries until the advent, and phenomenal growth, of Christianity. Nestled in the fertile ground of a philosophy that presumed the overwhelming value of human life, the Christianized Hippocratic model of medicine flourished.

While neither Christianity nor Hippocratic
medicine brought paradise, the ideal, a standard,
was established. The ideal was expected. Over the
centuries, it came to the point where people could
actually trust a physician to be interested solely in
their healing.

There were forces, however, that worked hard
(as always) to defeat the overwhelming influence of
Christian morality in the West; but, by and large,
the general ideals and principles held.

Scenarios like the one at the beginning of this
chapter would have been utterly rejected nearly any-
where, at least until the turn of this century. Until
rather recently, the oath *meant* something. While
its wording contained the ancient appeals to pagan
gods, the principle of protecting life was preserved.
Today, the oath isn't even *taken* by physicians, nor
is any alternate oath which explicitly prohibits killing.

Now, Dr. Jack Kevorkian kills "patients" with
apparent impunity. Oregon voters, in 1994, passed
the world's first law allowing doctor-assisted suicide. Abortionists proudly advertise in the yellow
pages. Hospitals go to court for the "right" to kill
medically dependent people against their will (as we
shall see later in this book).

What is happening here? Is this an aberration?
How did we get to this dreadful place from where
we were? Can this bizarre behavior by doctors be
stopped? I pray that, as in the past, the Church can
rise to the occasion and bring an end to this peril-
ous predicament. But first, we must understand
where we are.

Intent

Before launching into the remainder of the book, one issue must be emphasized—intent. This is central to our discussion. The great moral shift we have seen over the last thirty years has resulted in a shift of intent on the part of many medical people when it comes to the dying, the elderly, the infirm, and the nonresponsive.

Once, the intent may have been to provide medical care to assist a person in recovery from or stabilization of a condition—or, in the dying stages, to provide physical comfort and freedom from pain. However, now that intent may be to cause death. The distinction is important because one doctor, acting under the first intent (to care) may omit a treatment which will only exacerbate the condition to be treated. Another doctor may withhold a treatment merely to hasten death.

Throughout this book, when I speak of deathmaking by medical staff, I am not referring to the former kind of decisions, but the latter. The intent of the doctor, when you face such a decision for yourself or others, will not rest on the surface. That is, you will not know simply by what a nice person the doctor is whether his intent is to kill or cure. Therefore, it is the purpose of this book to help you become skeptical of orders to withdraw or withhold any ordinary or extraordinary care. You must treat such things the same way you treat the "presumption of innocence" in a court case. There must be a presumption of life and a presumption that such a withdrawal or withholding may be intended to kill. Make medical staff prove "beyond a reasonable doubt" that this move is in the best interest of the patient—and his continued life.

If medicine was what it once was—a Christian ministry—we might have reason for a lower standard. But, such is the world we live in.

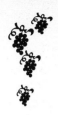

Chapter Two

"Brain Dead" Is Not Dead

Marie Odette Poole was dead in the eyes of most people. She was dead, but she carried a living child. For seven weeks after Poole had collapsed in the San Francisco elementary school where she taught, she was listed as "brain dead." But, though in a condition the public regards as dead, she continued to nurture her baby for almost two months.

The child, Marie Odette, was born alive on 30 July 1986 without complications and through a Cesarean section. After that, the life support system that assisted mother Marie, thirty-four, to breathe was disconnected, and the mother who had been "dead" for two months died.[1]

The story above should raise a lot of questions. First, do dead people carry their babies to term? If Marie was dead after she collapsed, what was she after the life support was disconnected? Double dead? If she was dead, why would she need *life* support? If Marie had recovered from brain death, would it be construed as resurrection?

Among the greatest successes of the Thanaphiles in recent times has been to convince the public—

and perhaps, themselves—that brain dead is dead. A long-time Thanaphile, Willard Gaylen wrote of brain death: "The problem (of euthanasia) is well on its way to being resolved by what must have seemed a relatively simple and ingenious method. As it turned out, the difficult issues of euthanasia could be evaded by redefining death."[2]

This "ingenious method" certainly worked well. In my experience, even most Christians acquiesce to removing life support (active euthanasia) if someone is brain dead. Perhaps this is because they do not fully understand the issues. Some of the issues involve questions like, "When is someone alive?" and "What does it mean when we allow someone to die?" These are questions we will address later, but one question we must answer here is the reverse of the first one, "When is someone *not* dead?"

Someone who is not dead is, by definition, alive. It is not necessary to know what constitutes life if we know that someone is not dead. The Christian ethic, and common sense, *presume life is present.*

Allow me to give two illustrations. If you are hired to demolish a building and you are *pretty sure*, as opposed to *absolutely* sure, no one is inside as you are ready to begin crashing in the walls, what do you do? Even if you have already checked out the building, you do so again. Why? Because you presume life is present. You would want to be absolutely sure that no one was inside before you started to demolish the building.

Suppose you see a person floating face-down in a swimming pool and you pulled him out. To all appearances, the man is dead. The skin is blue, you can feel no pulse, and you see no breathing. But, you start first aid procedures and call an ambulance, not the coroner. Why? Because you presume life is present. If there were any actual evidence of life, you would be obligated, in both cases, to be much more vigorous in presuming life.

A person who is brain dead may be assisted by as little life support as a ventilator—commonly called a respirator. This means that the heart, liver, kidneys, and the oxygenating capacity of the lungs are all working. If nothing else, these are irrefutable signs of life. So, beyond the mere presumption of life, there is evidence which commands response.

There are thirty different sets of criteria by which the medical profession may determine this misnamed condition. One of the most commonly used, the Minnesota Criteria, first laid out in a 1971 *Journal of Neurosurgery* article established that it does not even call for the measurement of brainwaves with an electroencephalogram (EEG);[3] nor do the British Criteria.

Both of these test for various responses to stimuli such as ice water in the ear or pin pricks on the soles of the feet. If there is no response to these simple tests the person is declared brain dead.

So, by these two most common methods of determining brain death, no one will even bother to check if there are brain waves. All of the commonly used criteria require the person to need a ventilator before he can be declared brain dead. However, if his heart is still beating and lungs still oxygenating the blood, that means that at least a part of his brain—the brain stem—is still functioning. Knowing this, the very idea of brain death is in question.

Often, the term *brain dead* is used interchange-
ably with *comatose*, but there are important distinctions—the presence or absence of a ventilator, for
example. Many are said to be brain dead just because the medical staff are not aware of the distinctions or the criteria. Overdoses of barbiturates and
other drugs can mimic brain death for as long as
forty-eight hours.

What all this means is that a person whose heart
is beating and whose lungs are still exchanging
oxygen for carbon dioxide and whose brain is still
functioning—even if only minimally—is defined as
dead (e.g., brain dead) solely because we cannot
prove consciousness or have them respond to us the
way we wish. Afterwards, we kill the dead person
and divide up any useful parts of his body for the
use of others. In essence, what brain death proponents are saying is that when medically dependent
people do not respond in ways we want them to,
they are worthy of death.

Paul Brophy, a fireman who was declared brain
dead in 1983, was "allowed to die" of starvation and
thirst by court order in the case of *Paul Brophy vs.
New England Sinai Hospital.* Brophy, however, did
not even fit the entire scope of brain death criteria.

> On July 7, 1983, during a neurological con-
> sultation, Brophy did not respond to verbal
> stimuli, but when something pained him,
> his right eye opened at times. When pres-
> sure was put on his breastbone, there was a
> "slight but appropriate movement in both
> upper extremities." A pin prick to the soles
> of his feet resulted in the withdrawal of both
> feet.[4]

Some relatives claimed that Brophy had said he would not want to live "that way"—that is, hooked up to a machine. However, only the lower court inquired as to whether Mr. Brophy would have wanted to die "that way"—that is, of starvation and thirst.

So, you might ask, "Why all the rush? Why would someone want to declare a living person dead before their time?" The answer is often simpler than one might suppose: money. Money saved in "useless" medical procedures, and, perhaps, money made on selling the "service" of procuring the body parts of the brain dead.

Another part of the answer comes down to the earlier quote by Willard Gaylen. There is a *deliberate* plan to have euthanasia become accepted by society. Knowing that the idea of killing sick people could not be easily sold to a people who still had vestiges of Christian ideas, it was found that redefining things (deception) would serve just as well.

Dying Is Not Dead

In the emotion-laden argument over death, it is important to remember that *dying* does not mean *dead*. Simply put, a dying person is alive until he is dead. This means we have all the responsibilities due to him that we would have toward any other living person. We also may have some additional responsibilities toward him because of his condition—relieving pain, providing comfort, and so forth.

If the person is both brain dead and dying, we have an obligation to protect him from the Thanaphiles who would "assist" his death. Of course, many brain dead people are not dying at all, though some doctors may wish to imply that they are. People have remained brain dead for many years without dying. Some have even recovered. But, the synonym for *brain dead* and *dying* is *alive*. We cannot treat these people as dead—or allow others to do so.

More of the Living "Dead"

Once consciousness is gone, the person is lost. What remains is a mindless organism.
—Stuart Younger, a psychiatrist at Case Western Reserve Medical Center

Younger proposes what is called the "cognitive" definition of death. That is, when a person loses his ability to think, he is dead. Such a definition includes any of those defined as brain dead, as well as the comatose, and even people in advanced stages of Alzheimer's disease or severe cases of Down's syndrome. This interpretation has become very popular among the Thanaphiles.

Dr. Joseph Fletcher of *Situation Ethics* fame, and highly regarded as a philosopher on medical ethics, has said that people with an IQ of twenty—and maybe anything less than forty—should not be considered persons.[5] These "philosophers" may seem to be only talking among themselves, but it is that same group who eventually end up in charge of the medical ethics boards of major hospitals.

What Is Death?

Robert Olive was a thief, and nobody likes a thief—particularly the man he is stealing from. Such was the case when Olive tried to break into a Portland, Oregon, apartment. The resident took umbrage and shot Olive in the face.

But, Olive survived the blast. I remember seeing him on television as he was being wheeled into Emanuel Hospital with an oxygen mask on his face and a reporter chattering away in the foreground. The purpose, however, of Olive's dramatic, televised entry into Emanuel was not for his treatment, but for the treatment of one Wesley Merrill, forty-four, who was several miles away in the Oregon Health Sciences University in need of a new heart. Olive had become a donor.[6]

What is wrong with this picture? The news report had said Olive had been declared brain dead within twenty-four hours of the shooting. Such statements are meant to soothe the listening audience because they have been trained to think of someone who is "brain dead" as dead.

But, something less obvious caught my eye. I was not watching the groomed reporter, but the man on the stretcher. He was wearing an oxygen mask! This was not a ventilator which assisted his breathing, but a simple mask giving a *breathing* man oxygen-enriched air.

This man was not dead! Yet, he was about to be made dead by the taking of the most vital organ in his body, his heart, which would be given to another. But, all of that was completely ignored, made irrelevant by virtue of the fact that this was to be Oregon Health Sciences University's first heart transplant. Olive was brain dead—and a thief, to boot—and his mother had given permission for the donation.

The definition of death, accepted by most states under the promotion of the Thanaphiles, is contained in the Uniform Determination of Death Act (UDDA). UDDA says,

> An individual who has sustained either 1) irreversible cessation of circulatory and respiratory functions, *or* 2) irreversible cessation of all functions of the entire brain, including the brain stem, is dead. A determination of death must be made in accordance with accepted medical standards. (emphasis added)[7]

Carefully note the *or* in this definition. Either section one or section two may be used to determine death. Part one is relatively simple and acceptable to even the most critical observer. If blood flow (circulation) or breathing (respiration) have stopped and cannot be started, the person is dead. The slippery part is section two. To all appearances, this would seem to indicate that the "entire brain" would have to be completely shut down. But, that is not the case. When the definition talks of the "cessation of all functions" then goes on to say that the tests must be conducted "in accordance with accepted medical standards," it means that only a select few functions will be tested. The remainder will be regarded as peripheral functions.

Those "peripheral" functions may include: heartbeat, breathing, blood being oxygenated by the lungs, blood pressure, good blood circulation (as seen by the blanching color of skin when it is pressed with a return to pink or brown when pressure is released), excretory function (evidenced by the filling of the urine bag beside the bed), hormones release by various glands, response to stimuli (such as the tapping of a rubber mallet on the knee or ankle), and many more evidences that the central nervous system is still functioning.

The heart's operation is completely independent from all but a small portion of the brain stem—but it still indicates brain function.

Robert Olive demonstrates one of the paradoxes of the modern definition of death. Of the two allegedly equal definitions, one may be dead under one, and alive under the other. What's more, brain dead people, like Olive, are treated by medical staff as though they were alive. They turn them in their beds to prevent bed sores, take their blood pressure regularly, and use postural drainage to prevent pneumonia. Is this really a cadaver—a dead person? Do the dead have blood pressure? Worry about bed sores? Get pneumonia? Of course not!

Robert Olive was dead according to the second part of UDDA, but not according to the first. That is the irony. It is possible to be both dead and alive according to UDDA.

And, this is not the only problem with UDDA. All the talk about irreversible cessation of brain function is a smoke screen. When "irreversible" is used when referring to circulation and respiration, it is simple to prove that it is irreversible because the heart and lungs cannot be restarted and they start to physically deteriorate. This is not the case when UDDA talks of the brain; otherwise, the Thanaphiles who wrote this would not have objected to alternative language which would have

called for the "destruction"—in the medical meaning of the term—of the entire brain. Instead, they
rejected that definition. What they wanted was to
be able to test only for select functions and prog-
nosticate that loss of those functions could not be
reversed. However, numerous cases have proved
them wrong.

The *Isanti County (MN) News*, in January of
1977, reported that a fourteen-year-old girl who
was declared brain dead, and whose parents were
asked to donate her organs, awoke. Two months
later, she was completely off life support and teas-
ing her sisters.

The *Journal of Clinical Neurophysiology* (vol. 5,
no. 4, 1988, p. 354) reported that seven brain dead
patients recovered.

The *Seattle Post Intelligencer* told on 26 January
1989, of a nine-year-old boy in Wichita, Kansas,
who was taken off life support. He recovered after
Dr. E. Abay had said "There was no brain
function . . . three or four times we'd see the pulse
go down to zero—no circulation at all to the brain
for thirty minutes on end . . . no one comes back
from this situation."

The same paper reported nearly one year later
on a Yakima, Washington, woman whom doctors
said was in a state of "cerebral death" emerging
from a deep, five-month coma, two to three days
after delivering her baby, Simon.

New Jersey Right to Life News reported in their
Euthanasia Edition of 1990 that the sound of a
grandson's voice apparently woke seventy-nine-year-
old Harold Cybulski in the Ottawa Civic Hospital

on 22 January 1989. The family was solemnly gathered in the hospital room while life support was disconnected and a priest prepared to give last rites. A curious grandson, Jeffery, who waited outside, peeped around into the room and cried "Grandpa!" Grandpa awoke. Two weeks later, he was released from the hospital and a month later, he bought a new car, and today drives around visiting family members. Quite a bit of activity for a dead guy.

And, according to the *Kansas City Times* of 28 September 1978, a nineteen-year-old Austin, Texas, man was declared brain dead and was being kept alive on a ventilator to "preserve his organs for transplant" while they searched for a matching organ recipient when the neurosurgeon noticed brain activity. On 13 February 1975, this same paper had noted that the wink of an eye saved S. William Winnogrond just as a surgeon was preparing to remove his kidneys and eyes for transplant.

Just two days after a doctor had asked Jennifer Keough's parents to donate her organs, the girl scratched out a message, "I wat to tak to my mom," according to the *Modesto (CA) Bee* (19 October 1989). When her mother arrived at Jennifer's Hollywood, Florida, hospital room, the young girl wrote notes to her. Her ventilator prevented her from speaking.

I could give more examples, but if brain death were truly death, these incidents could only be described as resurrections—miracles most Thanaphiles would be reluctant to acknowledge.

None of these people fit the first UDDA definition of death, but all of them fit the second. All of them were judged "irreversible." If any of them had fit the first definition, cessation of blood flow and breathing, they would have also fit the second (and then some). But, as it was, they fit only the second definition. What does that tell you about the accuracy of the second UDDA definition of death?

Alone, the second definition is merely a description of a condition that exists, not a criteria for determining death. That condition exists with all dead people, but quite a few living people as well. In fact, medical advances have been made in treating this condition of low or no apparent brain function and bringing about more recoveries.

Normally, the only treatment for death is burial. But if brain dead were actually dead, the medical profession would not be treating the condition. Thus, the brain dead condition has created a medical double-mindedness. There are people who are thought of as dead, but treated as if they were alive.

What Is Life?

The life of the flesh is in the blood.
—Leviticus 17:11, 14

Pity the poor deluded souls who believe that the Bible is only meant to be truth when dealing with moral issues, but not with scientific things. Almost daily, we hear of archæology and other sciences "discovering" what the Scriptures have said all along. Such is the case with this seemingly simple phrase from Leviticus written above. Note that it does not say that the life of the flesh is in the brain— or even in the heart or in the lungs.

God, the Creator of these bodies, clearly understood their operations. He, with this verse, captures the way the human body operates as an *integrated system*. The brain supplies some of the commands, but the heart operates on its own. The heart pumping and circulating blood does no good if the lungs are not breathing and oxygenating the blood. All the separate parts depend on the circulation and oxygenation of blood. Some parts clean the blood, others add nutrients, but all of them fail without oxygen carried to them by blood. The life of the flesh is in the blood.

In fact, this verse coincides very well with the first UDDA definition of death. If circulation or respiration (including both breathing and oxygenating) are irreversibly stopped, the person is dead. This is also the ancient understanding of death. Our detection abilities may be much more sophisticated and our technology may be able to assist these functions temporarily, but the facts remain the same.

The brain is not the central organ of life, as modern medical ethicists are proposing. Some people have suggested that this brain worship by modern scientists is a reflection of the humanistic pagan idea that the only difference between man and the animals is the ability to think. Therefore, they conclude, it is man's brain which makes him human and alive.

None of this, however, accounts for the "ghost in the machine," as some scientists call it. It is often called the mind-brain connection. They know there is something other than just a mechanism, a brain, behind human personhood. That "ghost" is the human spirit given by God which directs the "machine" of the brain. But, science is reluctant to admit the existence of a spirit.

Theological Implications

The brain death criteria for actual death falls woefully short of reality, but there is something behind the definition. The force of the brain death concept comes first from the man-as-animal belief. Then, the dehumanizing language comes into play. This is followed by a crude utilitarianism, a cost/benefit analysis, emerging when the arguments for acceptance of "brain death" are proffered. "He'll be nothing but a vegetable," some claim, perhaps not realizing that they have just dehumanized a person. Usually, the next words are something about the costs involved in "keeping him alive." Often, they mix their words with cluckings about the emotional burdens of the family in order to give them a sheen of compassion. But, there is no compassion for the brain dead. Willard Gaylen, quoted earlier, has cynically named brain dead people "neo-morts"—the new dead.

Christians, however, should recognize first, the *humanity* of the patient, then, their need. The response, according to Scripture, is obvious. To choose another path would be a profound departure from Christian teaching.

Certainly, there is no way for a Christian to agree with killing an innocent living person, even if he is called brain dead. Even the urgency advocated by doctors so that they might harvest the organs for transplant (an issue for another chapter) gives no justification for taking an organ from a living person who will die as a result of that removal. If the brain dead are not dead, then removing a vital organ from them while they are in this condition is nothing short of murder.

The taking of Robert Olive's heart was murder. He may have been a thief, but theft is not a death-penalty offense and did not warrant the theft of his heart. But, often, in the past, and, I am reminded, still today, Christians, even Christian doctors and other medical people, have been swept along by the current of today's medical ethics stream. Kept ignorant through euphemisms and obfuscation, Christian doctors and pastors have poorly advised people on the treatment of those labeled brain dead. But, as is true in all things, if we are disciples of His, we will know the truth and the truth will set us free. We just have to be willing to look at the truth.

What to Do

Reviewing the things we have discussed in this chapter, it is well to consider, in advance, how you might respond to something like this. You should be prepared should decisions about a brain dead person be up to you to decide. In fact, you should instruct others who might be in the position of making decisions about you if you are ever declared brain dead.

In such circumstances, the first rule is: Ask questions! Ask lots of questions, and don't stop until you understand everything and are completely satisfied. Remember, the person who is being called "brain dead" is a friend and is in *no* hurry to die. The only ones in a hurry are the medical staff. Don't let their anxiety affect you.

Questions you should ask about the declaration of brain death are:

> Who made the determination?
> What criteria did they use? Minnesota? Harvard? Their own special brand?
> What are *all* the *specific* tests that they used?
> Did they take an EEG? What did it show?
> Is the person's heart beating?
> Is he breathing or making an effort to breathe on his own?
> Do his lungs respire (exchange oxygen for carbon dioxide)?
> Are his glands producing hormones?
> Does his knee or ankle jerk when tapped?
> If pressure is applied to the skin, will it blanch and return to normal color upon release?
> Is urine being collected by a catheter?
> Does he have blood pressure?

If there is *any* response to any brain death test—regardless of which criteria are subscribed to—these are signs of life. Dead people *never* respond at all. If the answer is yes to any of the last questions, these are signs of life. None of these things are true of dead people.

If signs of life are present, it is your Christian duty to refuse any kind of stripping of his body parts or "pulling the plug" that will result in death. This is true whether the person has stabilized in the brain dead condition or is actually in the process of dying. He is alive and must be treated as such. It is up to you to watch over this person as you watch over your own life and insure that the social engineers don't carve him up or push him from brain dead to *real* dead.

Insist that all necessities—food, water, air, warmth, antibiotics, or other systemic support medications—be provided at all times, even to the dying. If any care has a chance of being effective in the curative sense, insist on it as well.

Don't let the medical staff get away with referring to the person with dehumanizing terms like vegetable (or even vegetative) or to talk around the patient as if he were not present. We have no idea what goes on in the mind of someone who is labeled brain dead or comatose. We don't know what level of consciousness exists. There are no objective scientific tests to measure that. So, you must treat these people as people. Talk to them. Tell them jokes. Tell them the news—national, local, and family. Read their favorite parts of the paper to them—sports, comics, national news, letters to the editor. Read books to them—the kind they liked before becoming too ill to read. Read the Scriptures to them. If they are conscious at all, they will appreciate being treated like live persons. It will show them that you haven't abandoned them and are out there to help and protect them.

I remember the time when I visited a fellow worker from my old job with the Parks Department who was on a ventilator and had been declared brain dead. I had witnessed about Jesus Christ to him on a number of occasions, but he'd always rejected it.

But, on my last visit with him, I just assumed that he was still there and I told him about the love of God again and pleaded with him to make peace with God through the cross of Christ. I don't know what happened inside him, but he died the following day. Perhaps I'll see him when I meet my Lord. I had to give him one more chance.

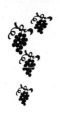

Chapter Three

Comatose Is Not Dead Either

Although Nancy was comatose, she waved at the camera, smiled when the nurses entered the room, and cried when visitors left.

Unfortunately, being comatose in today's medical America can get you dead—and not just brain dead, either. Many people have a distorted view of what the word *comatose* means. Most picture someone in a deep, unawakening sleep. It is not the same as brain death. The fact is that there are many kinds of comatose states, ranging from a kind of stupor-like wakefulness to a nearly permanent sleeplike condition.

Nancy, mentioned above, is Nancy Beth Cruzan. For years after her automobile accident, she lay in a bed or sat in her wheelchair in the Missouri State Rehabilitation Center smiling at the nurses who came in, crying when visitors left, and occasionally waving at people. She was fed by a stoma feeding tube—not because of an inability to swallow, but for the convenience of the staff. Nancy, it seemed, preferred one type of formula over another when she had the opportunity to taste them.

On 14 December 1990, circuit court Judge Charles E. Teel, Jr., signed Nancy's death warrant, permitting Missouri State Rehabilitation Center to stop feeding her. On 17 December, Joseph Foreman, a cofounder of Operation Rescue, and eighteen others, including two nurses, tried to enter the center and feed Nancy. All were arrested. Nancy, unaware of the attempt to save her life, continued to starve.[1] She starved to death on the day after Christmas.

The story was national news, so the Thanaphiles, in an effort to soothe already sleepy consciences, arranged for a public television crew to videotape her demise. It was all so peaceful. Nancy, under the hazy influence of dilantin and sedatives, looked like she was having a euthanasia—a "good death."

Measuring Up

Medical people have a scientist's need to measure things. They like to quantify what they see. In this light, it is not surprising that there are various scales to measure the level of coma that a patient is in. The most widely accepted is the Glasgow Coma Scale which rates comatose states by numbers arrived at by the responses of the patient to various stimuli.

Comas range from people who appear merely dazed but awake to the classical vision of the never-waking sleeper and everything in between. Generally, after the deepest kind of comas continue for more than three months, the person is said to be in a "persistent vegetative state" or PVS. The designation is more than unfortunate—it is dehumanizing.

Being nonresponsive does not make one a "vegetable" or even like a vegetable.

Barbara Blodgett, twenty-four, was one of those in a deep coma. Doctors even described her state as "cerebral death." But, she was also pregnant. The coma persisted from her accident on 30 June 1989 until 9 December—just over five months—when she gave birth to an eight-pound boy, Simon. As soon as the delivery was accomplished, she began to revive from the comatose state. Within five weeks of the delivery, Barbara was on her way home and continuing to recover from the coma and the brain stem injury that caused it. Barbara's father, Gregory Valenzuela, said, "I think the whole time she's been injured, she's been aware. She's just had no way of relating that back to us."[2]

Nor is she the only one of her kind. In 1991, thirty-year-old Debbie Chaltry gave birth while in a coma. She also began to recover after the birth.[3] Dead people don't have babies. Nor do they recover after having those babies.

The Glasgow Coma Scale[4]

Surprise the doctor—calculate the level of coma that your neighbor is in and *tell the doctor* what condition the patient is in. Keep in mind, though, that this scale is not to be used on children or those who are intoxicated, and certain kinds of injuries (spinal, for instance) will make the scoring invalid. But, where appropriate, the test is simpler than you might suppose. The scale runs from three through fifteen, with fifteen being the lightest coma. The calculation takes place in three types of activities, and when the scores are added together, you have the scale.

For instance, let's say that your neighbor has been in a car crash and has severe head injuries. You go to visit him a few days after the accident when his condition has stabilized. When you get to the hospital, the medical staff warns you that he is in a coma. You expect a sleeplike state, but you find it is not that way at all. When you speak, he responds to your voice, but is confused. He gets four points for that. He opens his eyes pretty much only when people address him—another three points. He doesn't respond very well physically but withdraws his arm or leg from pain—another four points. This gives him a Glasgow score of eleven. You must be careful to take any medications or sedatives into account, but, all things considered, this neighbor is doing pretty well.

Glasgow Coma Scale

Activity	Score
Verbal Response	
None	1
Incomprehensible sounds	2
Inappropriate words	3
Confused	4
Oriented	5
Eye Opening	
None	1
To pain	2
To speech	3
Spontaneously	4

Motor Response

None	1
Abnormal extensor	
(extended arm or leg rigidity)	2
Abnormal flexor	
(bent arm or leg rigidity)	3
Withdraws	4
Localizes	
(responds with appropriate limb)	5
Obeys	6

The comatose state ranges from a completely nonresponsive, mute, immobile patient to one who is fully oriented and awake. All are breathing (with or without help) and have heartbeats and pulses.

Having completed that exercise, note the obvious. This person, even at a stage three on the scale, is *alive*. Make sure he has adequate food and water, that he is comfortable, and that he does not lack treatment for any ailment. Then, just like your brain dead neighbor, talk to him. Read to him. Pray with him. And, above all, protect him from the Thanaphiles. Remember that Nancy Cruzan, according to the known reports and a videotape of her in the hospital, rated at least a ten on the Glasgow Scale—a very good score—and they *killed* her.

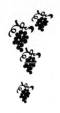

Chapter Four

Old and Infirm in America

I get no respect.
—Comedian Rodney Dangerfield

If this could be a theme song, it would be the theme song of America's elderly. Today's emphasis on youth excludes the elderly from consideration unless they are willing to publicly don the trappings and attitudes of youth. Notice the countless media features on old people who are "young at heart" and validate the sexually saturated, hedonistic pronouncements of the dominant paradigm.

The public loves youth and anything that reflects it. Whatever is old has to go—to be supplanted by the new. Old courtesies give way to new casualness. Old people have to be "progressive" to be taken seriously. For old people to cling to old ideas is, well, *old* fashioned and, *ipso facto*, bad.

Many cultures—even pagan ones—see the elderly as repositories of wisdom. This wisdom is what they are expected to produce for their societies. In America, the old are seen as useless. Especially useless are people who are infirm: the chronically ill, those with incurable illnesses or conditions, and the bedridden.

A great show is made of looking out for the disabled, but the less visibly disabled—especially those who constantly require expensive medical care—are only grudgingly tolerated. Listen carefully to the television debates over the health care crisis and hear how often "rationing" is mentioned, and you will understand just how dangerous it is to be elderly or infirm in America.

"Incurables" and "Defectives"

A Down's [syndrome child] is not a person.
        —Joseph Fletcher, noted medical "ethicist"

If the elderly, especially the sick elderly, are offensive to the bean counters and youth worshipers, those who are incurable or defective are positively loathsome. They remind us of the fragility of our lives and bodies in a way that we would rather not think about. The most commonly heard refrain is "I'd rather be dead than live like that!" It is surprising, however, how strong the pull of survival becomes when one is actually faced with that choice.

But, medical care for these people is often grudgingly given. The expense is carefully tallied and thrown into the equation. Included in the ranks of the incurables and defectives (and, yes, this last term is dehumanizing) are: diabetics, epileptics, those with cystic fibrosis, the mentally retarded, anencephalics, people with multiple sclerosis, AIDS, Alzheimer's disease, Parkinson's disease, Lou Gehrig's disease, chronic heart disease, high blood pressure, defective kidneys (needing dialysis), the mentally ill, and dozens of other crippling (and costly) conditions. These are on the hit list.

German physicians, even *before* the Nazis, were killing off "defectives" quite liberally with their T4 and 14f13 programs. Eventually, they were killing off young boys who had "poorly mottled ears." Death never says, "Enough!"

Money and the "Duty to Die"

Don't let young children suffer because of health care we give the elderly.[1]
—Richard Lamm, in an address called "The Ten Commandments in an Aging Society"

Richard Lamm, a former governor of Colorado, was not always this sensitive about the issue. He once, in speaking to a group of elderly people, said that the elderly have a "duty to die" and should save health care money for the young. And, he was not alone. While a brief tumult resulted from his famous "duty to die" speech, there was a surprising amount of public support in the media. Even those who thought his remarks crass spoke about how Lamm had "given us all some important things to think about."

According to author and *Washington Post* staff columnist, Suzanne Fields, in the mid-1950s, more than half of Americans believed that children should bear the burden of taking care of their aging parents. Thirty years later, less than 10 percent believed that.

This shift is clearly reflected in the treatment of the elderly we see today. It is more common now to have the elderly abandoned to nursing homes than to be taken in by family members—even when their care needs are minimal. *Parade Magazine* reported that unnecessary deaths of nursing home residents are frequent. "In California alone," the article said, "79 patients died between 1985 and 1986 as a direct result of mistreatment and neglect."[2] There are constant reports of over-medication for "pacification," assaults, thefts of patient property, and even experimenting with unapproved drugs without permission.

Medicaid is a staple of these places, but not nearly enough to provide anything like real care. Most states allocate only minimum wage payments (or just above minimum wage) for staff, which often leads to an untrained and even uncaring work force. Many reports exist of convicted felons working in nursing care facilities because the facilities have no way to check the backgrounds of workers. Abuses are understandable with such chintzy funding. It is a clear reflection of how we value the elderly that funding for such places is only enough to feed them peanut butter on bread and to have minimum wage attendants.

The whole socialized Medicare system is a tortuous maze of regulations designed to frustrate good care for the elderly, especially those needing nursing care. Homes are given a pittance to care for the patients and then prohibited by law to charge a private patient more than the state pays. The regulation is rarely followed. If it were, the home would close and many of the patients would receive no care at all.

Pharmacies that provide medications do so on the per-dose basis. The prices are fixed by bureaucrats. When a patient leaves or dies, the remaining medications are returned to the pharmacy, which in turn is supposed to reimburse Medicaid. Most do not. They resell the medications in order to recoup on the losses they incur from the fixed prices. Other ancillary services—labs, physicians, etc.—operate the same way. In the end, the people who make out the worst are the patients.

A friend, who worked for years as a nursing home administrator, has told me of how the state can get rid of troublesome patients by simply withholding obviously necessary medical care. One case she related happened in the mid-1980s to an elderly female patient with mild to moderate retardation. One day, she broke her dentures and refused to eat without them. My friend, the administrator, contacted the state about repair or replacement of the dentures and explained the gravity of the situation. Nursing homes are not allowed to force-feed patients. After several days of trying to coax the old woman to eat and several calls to her caseworker trying to get an exception for Medicaid to pay for the dentures, the patient was finally hospitalized. The nursing home staff asked the hospital to give the patient fluids through an IV. Ten days later, the hospital notified my friend that the woman was dead. She had refused the IV feedings, and the state, for want of two hundred dollars for the dentures, had let her starve to death.

Of course, one could always look at the cost/benefit analysis and say that if they had paid the two hundred dollars, she probably would have lived on for years—costing the state many thousands of dollars. Few would openly admit to such a motive, but, in cases like these, we are often told of the burden of life for people like this. But, that burden is, in reality, a financial burden on those who have the power of life and death over the unwanted of our society.

The "burden" of the elderly is that they cost money to keep around and they do not have anything that this society values anymore. Many of the elderly are rushed through court proceedings and declared incompetent. Sometimes, the elderly person is not even present at the hearing and does not have an attorney. A guardian is appointed to make all their decisions for them.

Winsor Smith, a Memphis State University professor who studied guardianship in thirteen states said that, if granted, guardianship reduces them to "wards of the court." They then have the status of legal infants who may no longer drive a car, vote, or in many states, hire an attorney. So, even if some object to the ruling, they cannot get an attorney to fight it for them. "A prisoner has more legal rights," Smith said.[3]

*Ration*ale for Abuse

Anyone who was awake during the debates over health care sponsored by the Clinton administration in 1993 had to have noticed the curious avoidance of the word *ration* in association with what they were planning. But, rationing was precisely what any publicly funded health care would, of necessity, entail. Even plans that only seek coverage for the poor must ration health care. In Oregon, we have a "model" health care plan that is supposed to insure that all Oregonians are covered by health care. And they are—if they suffer from the problems listed as the most necessary or if their incomes are at the lowest end of the poverty scale.

Naturally, the list was politically oriented. Near the top is treatment for alcohol and drug addictions. Abortion, an *elective* surgery is covered. But, try to get help if you have something that is not on the "approved" list and you'll find that the liberal politicians who drafted this law become curiously short of their famous "compassion." Try having a *chronic* illness, like cystic fibrosis, that recurs often and needs aggressive treatment, and you'll find yourself in a long line waiting for a short shrift.

The Clinton proposal would have been even worse. If your problem fell outside the list or if the treatment that actually worked was not listed, it would have been a *federal crime* to pay for or provide that treatment. But, nothing here suggests that there is not already rationing. Of course, "money" automatically rations medical care in the same way as it rations who gets the new Rolls Royce and who gets the 1979 Ford. There isn't much that can be done about that—or even much that I would recommend doing about that. In fact, I believe that both personal medical care and charity should be a part of one's personal responsibility. One ought not to insist on medical care for themselves that they cannot pay for or, for others, that they are unwilling to support. However, when medical care is covered by insurance or other means, all legitimate treatment should be given.

However, government intervention into the medical profession already provides plenty of incentives to not treat people with chronic problems. Worse yet is the poor attitude of many doctors toward people who have chronic illnesses or conditions. Doctors have become accustomed to the idea that medical resources are scarce and that they—and only they—must monitor the allocation.

Dr. Wolf Wolfensberger notes, "Afflicted people offend the cultural deities of youthfulness, beauty, fun and escape from pain and suffering."[4] Back in 1988, Wolfensberger's magazine, *TIPS*, reported that leaders in the British medical profession were withholding life-prolonging treatments from the elderly in order to "stabilize health care costs."[5]

Northwestern Life Insurance Company (it is obvious what *their* interest would be) conducted a poll to find out what Americans think of rationing health care. The vast majority of people agreed with one of six rationing proposals. But, a closer look reveals that Americans polled say they want to ration the health care of *other people*, not themselves.

And, rationing is already taking place. Most health care insurance plans have rules already in place about who can receive what kind of medical services based upon age and health. They are not about to "waste" perfectly good health care on someone who is chronically ill, other than to provide care designed to make them comfortable.

More commonly, under the health care promoted by the insurance industry, people are submitting to new supersensitive genetic tests which may be causing "selective non-treatment" by health maintenance organizations (HMOs) looking to cut costs. These genetic tests look for "markers" which may indicate the future likelihood of certain diseases and conditions such as certain cancers, Lou Gehrig's disease, Alzheimer's, cystic fibrosis, and many others.

HMOs are designed to cut costs wherever possible—which is good—but often this is done at the expense of giving good care. Doctors who are more careful and run a few more tests than the others in the HMO will find themselves pressured to cut back on "unnecessary" services or be ousted altogether. Providing "too much" care for the chronically ill may put one on a fast track out of an HMO.

A number of states have made it illegal for employers and insurance companies to require genetic testing because it was being used to discriminate against people who had a propensity—no matter how small—toward expensive medical problems. Often, the employers and insurance companies had misunderstood the significance of the tests and effectively blacklisted people who had little or no chance of developing the problem for which they had a "marker." So, it wasn't just those who truly were at risk for certain conditions who were discriminated against, but others as well. This injustice is not about drawing neat little lines—it eventually hurts everyone.

But, the prohibition against *requiring* the testing had little effect if the tests were already part of someone's medical record—or became part of their medical record when they went to their HMOs. Some people, aware of this possibility, have chosen to get such tests privately and at their own expense so that the results do not show up in their other

medical records.[6] The exception to this is the only
virus with civil rights—HIV. Records of it may only
be passed on if you specifically sign for them to be.

If you are one of those being frozen out of certain treatments, chances are, you will never know it.
You would never even be offered the treatment.
This is a direct result of the shift of the doctor's job
from being a healer interested in the patient, to
being a keeper of the sacred medical resources.

The Land of the Lost Medical Resources

"Beat the Reaper" was a hilarious skit by a 1960s
comedy troupe, Firesign Theater, which parodied
television game shows. In the skit, an individual
was injected with a disease and was given thirty
seconds to "name that disease" in order to be administered the antidote. The contestant, "under the
strict supervision of the director of the Armenian
Medical Association," was given the injection of
"Symptom Six—that *really big* disease." But, he failed
to identify the ailment and . . .

In 1994, Dutch television began broadcasting
"A Matter of Life and Death," in which a studio
audience votes on which of two patients on the
show will receive much needed, life-saving medical
treatment. The Dutch Ministry of Health, which
put on the show, claims that the show is intended
to stimulate debate on ways to control health care
spending.[7] Considering that the socialistic Dutch
health care system is the model for government
health care that many cite, it is interesting to note
that this cradle-to-the-grave system of complete care
may have to prevent some cradles and bring about
some early graves in order to keep itself financially

afloat. But, more ominous, this points out the essential premise of the Thanaphiles—that there is a limited pool of medical resources out there from which all medical help is drawn.

It may be true that, if a hospital has only ten ventilators (for instance), eleven people cannot be ventilated in that place, but this does not mean that all ventilators everywhere are in use. No one suggests that any medical facility offer services it does not have, but no one should be denied use of an existing ventilator on the chance that someone "more worthy" might later arrive. Nor should an old and sickly patient be removed from one because a young and otherwise hearty patient needs it. The ventilator on the older, more sickly patient is not a "lost medical resource"; it is saving a life. In general, the principle should hold that the doctor takes care of the patient in front of him—first come, first served.

But, this is not the attitude we see reflected today. People are seen as competing for medical resources, and the winners are declared by medical ethicists whose criteria is youth and usefulness. Yes, there are limited medical resources, if that's how you want to define the fact that there are only a finite number of medical personnel, hospital rooms, or life support devices. But, there is nothing resembling any kind of pool of resources that is capable of being allocated properly.

The men, rooms, and machines exist where they do. If more are needed somewhere else, new ones should either be built by those desiring them or existing ones should be moved from places where too many exist. Don't say, "There are only one hundred of these in the state, so I'll refuse old Mr.

Jones so that one will be free if we need one." You need one *now*—for old Mr. Jones!

There are, of course, times when medical resources must be rationed. During war or a natural disaster, there may be simply too many people to effectively treat at one time. The army medical unit with only four surgery tables may have to pick and choose who is first on those tables. The lesser injuries which still may require surgery will be put at the end of the line—as will those whose injuries are so severe that they will most likely die even if they receive the surgery. Those with the worst *survivable* injuries will be cared for first. This process is called triage.

Proponents of health care rationing usually point to triage as an example of what doctors should be doing every day across the entire country. The problem is that, in order to have triage, the doctor must have up-to-the-minute and total knowledge of the resources available, at least in his own community. But, doctors have no such knowledge or expertise.

More than that, the goals are completely different. The social triage recommended by the Thanaphiles is based upon the *social usefulness* of the patient and, thus, the patient's *worthiness* to receive treatment. But, notice that the goal of true triage—despite the emergency status—is not to weed out the "useless" but to save the maximum number of people regardless of their "worthiness." And, there is nothing akin to a battlefield emergency in normal medical practice today—at least not one that covers our entire society. There is nothing that would require the kind of rationing envisioned by the promoters of socialistic health care either. While the triage argument bubbled below the surface of the debate, there was an underlying inconsistency to the idea. The proponents wanted everyone to have health care—even if that meant less health care available for everyone.

Perhaps one of the strangest events of 1994 for me occurred during the great health care debate conducted in the media over the Clinton socialized medicine proposals. Many of the plan's supporters pointed to Canada as a model for the idea. Even Canadians with financial resources who often come to the U.S. for their medical care so they won't have to wait for crucial treatment, touted the Canadian system. But, the strangest thing I heard in the midst of that debate was when a proponent of socialized medicine actually complained that there were more CAT scan machines in the state of Oregon than in the entire nation of Canada! This man's defense of Clinton's health care was that medical resources should be more scarce at a time when people are receiving fatal nontreatment because of a purported existing lack of resources. According to this man, the CAT scan machine, which has been invaluable in saving so many lives, should have been less available. If people like this get their way, who do you think will *not* be on the short list to get CAT scans?

Future Triage

Search and destroy testing
—Prolife term for prenatal testing for Down's syndrome, spina bifida, and other conditions.

Amniocentesis and chorionic villi sampling
(CVS) were developed to uncover defects in unborn
children. Both tests have significant failure rates in
detecting or mistakenly indicating problems, as well
as often resulting in injury or death for the child.[8]
Not surprisingly, the development and promotion
of these tests was largely aided by the March of
Dimes—an organization devoted to eliminating
birth defects. The group is also a strong promoter
of abortion. While most people thought that the
March of Dimes was researching ways to *correct*
birth defects, they, in fact, were on the trail of ways
to make sure the "defectives" were never born. After
all, they were trying to stop *birth* defects, not *unborn* defects.

In other words, they wanted only nondefective
babies to come to term and be born. "Defective"
infants were to be destroyed before birth so as not
to spoil the average. With amniocentesis and CVS,
they began to move toward their goal of zero *birth*
defects. If, out of 1,000 pregnancies, for example,
three babies were tested and found to be "defective"
and aborted and 997 were born without defects,
that would mean a 100 percent rate of "curing"
birth defects. They could announce their great success in eliminating birth defects and brag that, without their efforts, three "defective" children would
have been born.

But, March of Dimes isn't alone in this concern. In 1986, California became the first state to
require such testing of all pregnant women. They
also have centralized genetic records. Women can
still refuse the test, but must sign a waiver of liability in order to do so. At the moment there is no

penalty for knowingly continuing a pregnancy with a "defective" child, but of what use is it for the state to record such tests out of concern for birth defects if they do not plan an attempt to reduce their numbers? When a woman signs that "waiver of liability," whose liability is being waived? Could the government later condition future state aid for a retarded child, for instance, if the mother refused testing or tested positive for Down's syndrome but didn't choose abortion?

With the current trend toward socializing medicine, those who refuse "treatments" like abortion could be sequestered from all medical help.

Dr. Neil Holtzman, an expert in genetic testing, said, "It is not out of the realm of possibility to use genetic testing, prenatal diagnosis and abortion as a means of reducing costs."[9] Only time will tell, but California's law is being eyed as a model for other states—and these movements do not tend to go backwards. Truly, these tests are "search and destroy." But, what is good enough for the unborn "defectives" is good enough for *you*.

Perhaps you've read about the Human Genome Project in the newspapers over the last few years. The science is extremely complex, but the moral issues are not. The project's goal is to map the human genetic material in such a way as to be able to locate the markers for human traits from eye color to temperament. They will locate up to one hundred thousand genes stretched out across the human DNA and label them according to their function or trait.

At the moment, some genes have been identified as markers for cystic fibrosis, muscular dystrophy, sickle cell anemia, cancer, and even a tendency toward alcoholism. But, there is no central map of the gene's structure. The Human Genome Project, if successful, would be the beginning of that ability. If the currently available ability to splice genes were tied to such knowledge, parents could almost design their own children by size, color, intelligence, appearance, natural abilities, and many other traits.

But, more dangerous today is the increasing ability to find markers that show tendencies toward heart disease, cancer, Alzheimer's disease, and dozens of other conditions. Some of the markers show a 100 percent probability of certain problems while most show much lower probabilities. If states follow the examples of Utah and California and develop centralized genetic records, who knows to what use such knowledge would be put.

While the German Third Reich may have been, in most minds, the ultimate example of the eugenic philosophy of ridding itself of "defectives," it is worth remembering that two years before Adolf Hitler enacted his first "hereditary health law," at least thirty U.S. states had legislation dealing with "hereditary defectives."[10] There were mass, forced sterilizations of such "defectives" in this country—a practice upheld in court by none other than liberal saint and "defender of civil rights," Oliver Wendell Holmes. American physicians like Foster Kennedy were viewed as trailblazers in eugenic theory—even by the German Nazis. So, one may not necessarily have to manifest a particular disease or condition anymore if the doctor discovers an inherited propensity toward that problem.

Could such information be used to deny someone a job? The "right" to marry and have children? Government benefits? Medical care? All these and as many more possibilities as an evil mind could imagine will be opened up—and used—if we let them.

Don't get me wrong. There are good uses for this knowledge. We cannot put this genie back in the bottle—nor should we try. Therapies have been, and are being, developed to actually treat genetic problems. But, the major push is toward getting rid of the "defective" people. Whether that continues is going to depend on our willingness to insist on Christian medical ethics across the board.

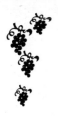

Chapter Five

"Pulling the Plug" and Other Plantation Favorites

On the first day, the old woman's mouth became dry and coated with thick phlegm. Over the next few days, her lips became parched and cracked. In the following days, her eyes sank back in their sockets and her cheeks became hollow. The mucous lining in her nose eventually cracked and caused a nosebleed. After a week, her skin became dry and scaly and hung loosely from her body. The woman's bladder was burning because her urine had become so concentrated. The drying out of her stomach caused dry heaves and her body temperature rose precipitously. The drying out of her brain cells would have caused convulsions had it not been for the paralytic drugs the doctors had administered to her. But eventually, all her major organs failed, including the lungs, heart, and brain, and she died. It had taken all of thirteen days. The doctors had compassionately "pulled the plug," and the old woman had died of thirst.[1]

"Pull the plug" sounds so innocuous. But, it is not. Those familiar with the issue of killing the infirm remember well the names of recent victims, like Nancy Cruzan, killed at age thirty-three in 1991;

Christine Bussalachi, killed by thirst at twenty in 1991; Nancy Ellen Jobes, thirty-two, killed by order of the New Jersey Supreme Court in 1987; Paul Brophy, "allowed to die" of starvation and thirst; and half a dozen others. But, these are only the handful whose names and circumstances become known to the public. Claire Conroy, eighty-four, the subject of one of these court-ordered starvation attempts, outfoxed the Thanaphiles by dying of other causes before they could "unplug" her. This was one of those rare instances of escape from the "compassion" of the Thanaphiles.

In the scenario above, repeated thousands of times a year in this country, a person is denied nutrition and hydration. The Thanaphiles say "nutrition and hydration" hoping you won't notice that those are just fancy words for food and water. The old woman above and those named below were killed with thirst and starvation and suffered the symptoms listed.

This is no mere "disconnecting." When one "pulls the plug," it is not like pulling the plug on a lamp where the light immediately goes out. Nor can this be called "allowing someone to die." Stopping a person from eating and drinking is not "allowing" something, but rather, a positive "acting upon" someone with the intent to kill them.

You might have noted that the old woman above was given a paralytic to stop her convulsions. This was not for her benefit. Dehydration is one of the most horrible ways to die that anyone can imagine. It is horrible to experience and horrible to watch. But, with a paralytic, the family, waiting for it to "be over," does not have to see the retching or convulsions, and they don't have to hear the person call out for water. It is all peaceful and serene as the object of their "compassion" dies a horrible death inside but dies with "dignity" outside.

To be fair, I must say that there are times when a dying patient cannot take food or water, even intravenously, without terrible discomfort. But, in such cases, the person does not die of the lack of water or food, but from the disease process itself. And, it is important to note that many people are being denied food and water who are not even dying, but merely comatose or incapacitated in some way.

What Are the Plugs?

When people talk of "pulling the plug," they are referring to the various kinds of life support mechanisms to which a person who is either dying or is in a stable, but dependent, state might be attached. "Pulling" the plug means to turn off or remove these mechanisms, thereby causing or "allowing" the patient to die. The most common mechanisms are as follows:

1) Ventilator—a machine, often erroneously called a respirator, which pumps air into a person's lungs at regular intervals, simulating breathing. The air may be regular or oxygen-enriched, depending on the need. It is used when the ability of a person to breathe is impaired by neurological damage, muscular inability, or weakness. This is probably the most common apparatus to which people refer when they talk about "being hooked up to machines."

2) Cardiopulmonary bypass pump—this is a machine which temporarily replaces the heart's pumping action while surgery on the heart is performed or while a patient with a degenerating heart is waiting for a transplant. Attempts to make a portable, mechanical heart which will last extended periods of time (or even for a lifetime) have, thus far, failed.

3) Pacemaker—a mechanical heart "shocker" which delivers a small electrical charge to the heart to stimulate the muscle contractions necessary to pump blood. Most of these are set up to only come into play when there is an arrhythmia—when the heart misses a beat or several beats. Some are set up to stimulate continuous beating.

4) Nasogastric tubes and stomas—the first is a small tube for feeding which runs down the nose into the stomach. Nutritional pastes and liquids (called "nutrition and hydration") are mechanically pumped through these into the stomach. The stoma is a larger tube which is surgically inserted into the stomach and exits through the skin just above the belly. The person eats by squeezing a tube of nutritional substance directly into the tube.

These devices are put in place under a number of conditions. The person, because of neurological or muscular damage, may not be able to swallow. The patient's esophagus may have been cancerous and removed. Or, it may be simply easier on the nursing staff to feed the patient this way than to take the time necessary to spoon-feed someone unable to feed himself. This was the case with Nancy Cruzan.

5) Intravenous (IV) needles—an IV is inserted into virtually *every* patient who is admitted into a hospital. It is used to deliver hydration (water) and various medications. Sometimes, it is used to deliver nutrition for people who cannot receive it in other ways.

6) Treatment—includes everything from chemotherapy to antibiotics and surgery to cleansing wounds. This is medical care extended for any kind of illness, injury, or condition. Under normal circumstances it is called treatment, but for the dying, comatose, and "brain dead" it is often called futile and regarded as "life support."

7) Palliative care—pain relief.

These are the things most often included under life support, especially when people are talking about those who are in the dying process or, in some way, unable to respond. It is important to understand what each of these things are and what they entail. When faced with the circumstance, one should always determine exactly what things a doctor is talking about when he says that someone is on life support.

We're All Together in This

If you think about it, we are all on life support. We all need food, water, warmth, and air. Under most circumstances, when a doctor talks about life support, he is implying that it is extraordinary care and might be stopped. But, let's take a look at some kinds of life support we have listed and see just how unextraordinary they are.

What does the ventilator do? It supplies air. We all need air and most of us have had an occasion to know just how it feels to be short of it. It is a supremely unpleasant experience. But, a ventilator seems so "extraordinary"—so *mechanical*. However, think for a moment how "extraordinary" a pair of crutches, or mechanical arms, or wheelchairs are. All of them are machines that replace a capacity a person has lost. Either through neurological damage or just plain weakness, a person's body is unable to raise his own chest and draw breath. Is this a reason to die if we are able to help him? A ventilator is a relatively simple regulated pump which, in some circumstances, uses an oxygen enrichment system. They are uncomfortable and hard to live with. (I know, I've spent some time on one.) But, as they say, the alternative is much worse. Wheelchairs and artificial limbs cannot be exactly comfortable or easy to live with. But, they have gained acceptance.

There are individuals, probably in your own town, who work and live with a ventilator day in and day out. They carry around what is called a "turtle," which is nothing more than a portable ventilator. Ed Roberts, forty-two, who had polio when he was young is quadriplegic (has little or no use of all four limbs) and has such a device on the back of his wheelchair. He flashes at the phrase "victim of polio" because he refuses to be a victim. His determination has caused him to pave the way for the disabled to attend the University of California at Berkeley. He is the father of a young boy and the originator of the "curb cut" that we now see at curb corners across the country.[2] But even if he weren't so determined (and successful), should he still be a candidate for "pulling the plug?"

Imagine being deprived of air. Even when someone is comatose or "brain dead," it is possible that they feel that deprivation. They usually *act* like they feel it when "unplugged" by thrashing around (unless they've been given paralytics for the benefit of the family). The comatose or brain dead person who resurfaces from their long trip to who-knows-where often reports having heard the conversations of doctors and family. Barring any evidence that the person does not feel the effects of starvation and thirst, we should assume that they do.

The truth is, just because they don't respond to us the way we would like, that does not mean there is nothing going on inside. We have no way of knowing what these people are thinking.

The cardiopulmonary bypass pump and the pacemaker serve similar functions. But, the pump actually pumps the blood, often while surgery is being performed on the heart. The pacemaker, by means of electric shocks, keeps the heart itself beating regularly. Neither is a long-term solution, but both are vital to bridging the gap. To shut off either of these is to essentially create a heart attack and to kill someone. It deprives the heart of oxygen, causing the muscle of the heart to die. As one whose heart has done this, I can testify that this is very painful.

The key to understanding this situation is that so long as the lungs are taking oxygen and putting it into the circulating blood and removing the carbon dioxide and expelling it, the person is alive. Part 1 of the UDDA we discussed in an earlier chapter says the irreversible absence of these is death. But, the corollary is, if a machine *will* reverse these, the person is not dead. The heartbeat is necessary—

even when artificially maintained. Many live out
their daily lives with pacemaker devices. Many have
been placed on cardiopulmonary pumps (as I have)
so that bypass and other heart operations like artificial valve replacements can be done. If we think
the pump is too artificial, what about the plastic
and stainless steel valves that keep thousands alive
today? The fact that some assistance is mechanical
does not make the life itself artificial.

But, probably the most controversial life support is artificial feeding through a tube or IV. Most
people don't realize it, but it has become nearly
universally accepted in the medical field that food
and water, when delivered by tube, is medical treatment as opposed to ordinary care. Can you compre-
hend that? The word *treatment* usually refers to a
means of combating an illness or condition. Yet
now, what we do every day to nourish our bodies is
considered medical treatment.

What is used to confuse the issue here is that
the *means* of delivery is unusual. But, there are people
who live and work every day in offices and factories
who feed themselves through stoma tubes into their
stomachs. If you want to get technical, using a fork,
spoon, or drinking glass is as artificial as any tube.
Here, as discussed earlier, the euphemisms come
into play. Food and water are magically transformed
into nutrition and hydration.

Here in Portland, Oregon, we get our water
from the Bull Run Reserve about twenty-five miles
out of town. It starts in a huge, protected, enclosed
watershed area, where the water runs down into
Bull Run Lake. From there, it is controlled by a

series of dams and is sent by five-foot conduits to the city reservoirs, and, from there, to homes and businesses in Portland. When I worked for the water bureau, I actually worked inside some of those large conduits and did periodic cleaning inside huge artificial reservoirs and tanks. I worked in the pump rooms that supplied water to the west hills of the city.

It's funny that all of that equipment is in operation to deliver *water*. But, if that water passes through a six-inch plastic tube in a hospital it becomes unnatural hydration. A similar illustration could show the farming, processing, delivery, and sale of food which, when given to the medically dependent, becomes unnatural nutrition. Don't be fooled by these misleading terms.

Starvation and dehydration, as described earlier, result in a horrible death. Would it be any less frightening and torturous if you were deprived of eating with forks and spoons than if you were deprived of eating through a stoma? What it really boils down to is not the means, but the food itself. It is not the "artificial" thing that people are being deprived of when this particular "plug" is pulled, but the nourishing food.

The fact is that the "artificial" tube is *never* removed. It is left in place as a means of delivering paralytics, anti-convulsants, sedatives, and other medications to make watching someone die easier on the viewer. But, whether you eat with a fork or a stoma, if you are starved and dehydrated, you will end up just as dead. And now, it doesn't seem to matter if you make your wishes plain.

In 1995, eighty-three-year-old Marjorie
Nighbert died after two weeks of being deprived of
food and water. The issue under consideration was
never Nighbert's wishes. Everyone knew she wanted
to be fed and given water. The court, however,
determined that she was not competent enough to
ask for them.[3]

Another "plug" that is pulled is medical treatment—meaning medical treatments other than the
newly defined food and water. Treatments include
everything from kidney dialysis, which temporarily
or permanently replaces the function of the kidney
(cleaning the poisons from the blood), to simple
antibiotics. Surgical procedures which are remedial
are also in this list.

In late 1994, baby Ryan Nguyen was being deprived by the staff at Sacred Heart Hospital in
Spokane, Washington, of both kidney dialysis and
a simple remedial surgery to remove a bowel blockage. They had removed Ryan from dialysis without
the parents' permission and despite their repeated
demands that the treatment be provided. It took a
court order—after a dangerous thirteen-day denial
of dialysis—to get the hospital to resume treatment.
It took an emergency helicopter ride to another state
to find a hospital and a doctor willing to treat Ryan
like a living human being.[4]

Such instances are not new. Back in the early
1980s, in Bloomington, Indiana, a child only known
publicly as Baby John Doe was starved to death for
want of a simple procedure to correct an esophageal
atresia, a blockage in the esophagus (the pathway
from the mouth to the stomach). But then, the
child was a Down's syndrome child and the parents

hadn't bargained for that, so they gave their permission to apply the "non-treatment of choice" (a chilling image concerning what "choice" means in the abortion industry). He couldn't be fed because his esophagus was blocked, and his esophagus was blocked because he was denied a simple medical treatment. It took more than a week for him to die.[5]

A Baby Jane Doe was similarly killed for having the gall to be born with surgically correctable spina bifida.

In both cases, the children had no fatal illness or condition. But, in both cases, the courts supported the starvation orders based upon their parents' "right to privacy." The courts also upheld both sets of parents' "rights" to do this particularly cruel and gruesome postpartum abortion on their children—or should we just call them *fourth-trimester abortions?* (Do I hear *fifth* trimester, anyone?)

As you can see, the "progress" from these earlier situations to that of Baby Ryan is that the medical staff no longer thinks that the parents' right to privacy is sufficient. They believe that they should be able to decide on their own whether these children should get treatment, and they'll take you to court to assert their "right" to kill undesirable children. Nor are these isolated incidents. These are some of the very few that come to public attention. Thousands go unnoticed.

Often, when a person is elderly, extremely ill, comatose, or brain dead, the doctor will simply refuse to give the patient antibiotics when they come down with pneumonia (a common ailment among the elderly and bedridden), which will result in the patient's death. Along with such antibiotics, treatment is often needed to remove excess secretions from the lungs, especially where the lungs, through injury or condition, have a diminished capacity. If the secretions are not removed, the person literally drowns, very slowly, as the excess fluids build up within him. This is often done with the intent to "allow death"—a euphemism for "kill." In cases like these, a person who is not dying or has no end-stage terminal condition, and whose life is easily protected with a simple regimen of antibiotic treatment and lung drainage, is killed by neglect. They are "non-treated."

These, and many others, are ordinary courses of treatment. But today, they are only considered *ordinary* by many in the medical field for the fit and those who will "contribute to society." It is one thing to decide that a week-long course of antibiotics for a cancer patient expected to die in hours or days is futile. But, to decide that antibiotics for a comatose patient who is expected to live for years—and has no end-stage terminal condition—is futile, just because it will not bring him out of his comatose state, is nothing short of murder. The withholding of medical care in order to hasten the death of someone who is not dying is murder by malicious neglect.

The Myths of "Keeping People Alive" and "Playing God"

Someone can only be "kept alive" if they are alive.
—Julie Grimstead, Center for the
Rights of the Terminally Ill

While, to some, this may seem to be a simplistic statement, there is an incredible truth here. None of the life support techniques in medicine can keep a dead person alive. They may keep someone from dying and they may even briefly prolong the process of dying, but they never keep the dead alive. The difference is vast. If a person is comatose or brain dead, is not dying of any other cause, and needs, for instance, a ventilator, he will surely die from suffocation if he is not assisted in his breathing. The ventilator, however, will not prevent him from dying from any other fatal illness or condition. Remember, these life supports are only being applied to two kinds of people: 1) ones who have no fatal illness or injury and, 2) those who do, and who are quickly heading toward death. But, one word describes both groups—*alive.*

Most of the arguments that involve keeping people alive are predicated on the assumption that the person is actually dying from some illness or condition. Certain kinds of cancer are but one group of many recognized terminal conditions. But, one could also consider diabetes, cystic fibrosis, high blood pressure, and dozens of other conditions to be "terminal." All are incurable. All will result in the eventual death of the sufferer.

The difference is that those with, say, malignant lymphatic sarcoma (cancer) may have less than a year before the condition kills them; cystic fibrosis (present at birth) usually kills the afflicted by their early teens. Diabetes will definitely shorten life.

So, if we are going to talk of keeping people alive, let's consider taking the insulin away from the diabetic. Let's refuse to give antibiotic treatment and remove the excess secretions from the lungs of the one with cystic fibrosis. And, let us take the blood pressure medication away from those who we are "keeping alive" with daily doses of it.

I'm being facetious, of course, but it illustrates the point. Those we claim to be keeping alive are most often people whose comprehending eyes we do not have to look into while we tell them that we will be "pulling the plug" on the things they need to help them live. We only do such things to people whom we do not have to tell—the comatose, the severely retarded, the brain dead. But, there is one thing about this group that is identical to those receiving blood pressure medication, insulin, or antibiotics—they are all alive. They are just as alive as you are, and just as deserving of whatever assistance they can get to extend and enrich their lives. So, the provision of medical assistance has become discriminatory. Give it to those who are capable of asking for it and who will be "productive citizens" after they receive it. Deny it to people who have no ability to take care of themselves or defend themselves and to those who aren't cogs that help our great society run.

It used to be that only people who killed others without cause were accused of "playing God." Murderers, abortionists, and doctors who "put people out of their misery" were "playing God," not people who tried to help others. Is it "playing God" to perform cardiopulmonary resuscitation (CPR)? How about using first aid to stop massive arterial bleeding? Should you even dial 911? After all, you might be "playing God."

Suddenly, it is those who want to preserve life who are now accused of "playing God." Is God suddenly in the business of taking lives? Or, is God really sovereign over our time to die, and are we—not knowing all things—merely working to preserve life until it is God's decision for it to end?

Killing or Allowing Death

One of the soothing phrases of the Thanaphiles is "allowing people to die." It has the genteel sound of "letting nature take its course." The issue becomes more difficult in many people's minds when the phrase is used in connection with a person who is rapidly approaching death from some unalterable condition or incurable disease. In some cases there is truly an issue of allowing death.

A good example is the person in the last stages of cancer. It would be truly futile, and probably vastly uncomfortable, to attempt chemotherapy. It would be better to use palliative care (pain control) and make him as comfortable as possible. This, however, is not the time to deny food or water or air—the very substances of life—in a way that will shorten his life. Sometimes, people who are close to death cannot comfortably tolerate food, but some kind of nourishment and water must be provided, probably intravenously. There may also be cases where even these cannot be tolerated, but a decision to withdraw food and water should always be closely scrutinized. And, it goes without saying that one cannot "allow" someone to die who is not dying—as is the case with most comatose patients and brain dead people. Most of the "plugs" for pulling deliver one of the essentials of life. Ventilators and even cardiopulmonary pumps deliver oxygen. Feeding tubes and IVs deliver food and water.

One does not "allow" someone to die by depriving a person of any of these, regardless of the complexity of the means of delivery. Antibiotics are *ordinary* care for regular people or unresponsive people. Allowing one to die is only applicable to those who are actually dying.

Theological Implications

Feed the hungry. Clothe the naked. Comfort the afflicted.

These are universal and unilateral commands of Scripture. How could "feed the hungry" *ever* square with stopping food and water to any person—dying or not? How could "comfort the afflicted" ever square with imposing thirst torture?

The fact is that we are to help and care for those who are dependent. We can begin by not dehumanizing them. Try to imagine Jesus telling us, "Love your vegetable as yourself." Is it hard? Try "neo-mort" or "gomer" (medical shorthand for Get Out of My Emergency Room) in that sentence. The reason it is so difficult to say is that you instinctively know that these people are your neighbors, nothing less!

The pagan mindset may be to calculate their future worth to society and dispatch those who are what medical ethicist Daniel Callahan, director of the Hastings Ethics Center, called "biologically tenacious" (meaning that they just keep on living and won't die for everyone else's convenience), but we cannot think that way.

The pagan ethic, according to Callahan is that a "denial of nutrition may in the long run become the only effective way to make certain that a large number of biologically tenacious patients actually die. . . . Given the increasingly large pool of super-annuated, chronically ill, physically marginal elderly, it could become the non-treatment of choice."[6] Jesus said, "Feed the hungry." Which ethic will you follow?

What to Do

In the previous two chapters, we have discussed the worst-case condition of your friend or neighbor. I advised you to ask a lot of questions about the exact nature of his condition. This was not so much because it would change your decision to treat him as a real, living person, but to confirm to you that this person is truly living and to send a message to the medical staff that you *know* he is living.

So, now is not the time to ask questions about his condition. Now is the time to firmly demand that every type of life support needed to help the person live must be given. Ask questions about what any ordinary person might need under similar conditions. Would he need pain relief? Would he need a diet high in protein or other nutrients?

Once you assess the person's need, follow the Bible. Do unto others what you would have them do unto you—namely, feed the hungry, give drink to the thirsty, care for the afflicted, relieve pain wherever possible. Remember, you are making a decision for *somebody else*. You must assume that the person wants to live—no matter how that kind of life looks or feels to you. You don't have the right

to decide whether or not another wants to die. The
result is too permanent.

Then, you'll want to closely monitor the delivery of this life support. Some medical staff may
try—as in Baby Ryan's case—to simply shut down
life support without consent. So, set up a system
with friends and relatives to stop in on the person
at least once a day to talk to him and check on the
life support.

Learn what signs to look for to see that all the
support is still working and teach others to identify
those signs. Communicate with the friends and
relatives who are often involved. Also, remember
what I said earlier about talking to the person himself. In all your zeal to deal with the medical staff
and understand the truth about the condition of the
sick person, don't forget the person himself.

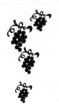

Unholy Sacrifices

The custom of human sacrifice admits that the life of one is taken to save the lives of many, or that of an inferior individual is put to death for the purpose of preventing the death of somebody who has a higher right to live.[1]

—Nigel Davies

Paganism doesn't change much. The technology and religious particulars may color it, but the same philosophy results in the same practices. One of those practices is human sacrifice.

Nigel Davies, author of *Human Sacrifice in History and Today*, hit the nail on the head in his descriptions of this most common of pagan practices. I say pagan because, in his exhaustive work on the practice, Davies, who seems to have no little sympathy for the custom, frankly admits that it was Christian missionaries who ended the practice. Continuing from the above statement, he says:

"Ritual killing often thrived in remote continents only until it was extirpated by people who were Christians."

Nor is he the only person to make that observation. An early 1900s book coauthored by a German lawyer and a German doctor called *Permitting the Destruction of Unworthy Life* promoted the taking of the lives of the handicapped and mentally retarded. The lawyer, Karl Binding, complained: "The long and painful development [of the idea of killing "valueless" people] over the centuries has been retarded partly because of the Christian way of thinking."

Author Garry Hogg noted in his book *Cannibalism and Human Sacrifice* that the practices were "in almost every part of the world, except Europe"[2] without noting that these things had been stopped by the Christianizing of Europe. Prior to that time, various groups of Europeans killed and ate their fellow man with as much vigor as any other group of people.

But now, I assert that much of the killing we are discussing in this book fits the category of human sacrifice as defined by Davies. In my former work on this topic, my coauthor and I defined human sacrifice this way: "The murder, torture, and/ or cannibalism of an innocent person justified as beneficial for himself, for another person or for society."[3]

After having studied human sacrifice modes throughout the world, Davies concluded: "The underlying conditions did not alter: lack of any benevolent redeemer, absence of a truly humane ethic, and, finally, belief in a ceaseless cycle of rebirth that turned the death of man into a trivial incident."[4]

These elements are present in our society today. There is no acknowledged redeemer. The humane ethic has been replaced by a cost/benefit analysis.

And, death has been made trivial by beliefs in either reincarnation or universal salvation (note the near-death experience pattern with no hell) or the belief in no afterlife at all.

The Bottom Line

Human life has economic value only as a function of his ability to produce goods and services that are demanded by others.

—Dr. Richard Baily

Does this sound like the doctor you want? No? Well, it may be like the doctor you already have. This sentiment is not isolated to a few, but has become the controlling ethic of medicine in America. It reflects the attitude that my own doctor had once, that would have denied me the opportunity for a life-saving treatment had he felt I wasn't going to be a "contributing member of society."

Other writers are equally blunt:

> Disparity between the needs of the health care system and human needs sometimes causes the sacrifice of human needs to the larger policy making structure. . . . From a cost/benefit viewpoint, society cannot benefit sufficiently enough from the limited future productivity of such persons to justify spending an increased amount of finite medical resources on them.[5]

Notice the use of the word *sacrifice* here. He says we are sacrificing "human needs," but, in reality, we are sacrificing human lives. And, unto what god do we sacrifice? "The larger policy making structure." Some god! Actually, the real god is described

in the second paragraph. The god is Mammon—
money!

But, that sounded too crass. So, the spin doctors and public relations men for the new ethic went
to work devising semantic gymnastics to cover their
motives. Out of it all came the phrase "quality of
life." There was a time when that phrase indicated
that we were seeking ways to remove bad *conditions*
to improve lives. Now it was to mean that we would
remove bad *lives* to improve conditions.

And, being scientific, medical science has longed
for a simple formula by which to determine who
should be "sacrificed to the larger policy making
structure." Eventually, some experimental physicians
came up with one, primarily for babies born with
spina bifida, though it could easily be applied to all.
The formula went like this, $QL = NE(H+S)$:
Quality of Life equals Natural Endowments (ability) times the sum of the contributions from Home
and family and the contribution from Society. If,
under this formula, you have quality of life, then
you live, if not, you die. Note: the rich (or well-
connected) always live because they can pay their
own way. But, people are being killed to benefit
others. The others, apparently, are more valuable
than those "inferior" people who are killed.

Remember the definition at the top of this chapter again. "The custom of human sacrifice admits
that the life of one is taken to save the lives of
many, or that of an inferior individual is put to
death for the purpose of preventing the death of
somebody who has a higher right to live." Doesn't
that describe what we are doing today?

Who Is Inferior?

One "inferior" group is the nonresponsive. Those who don't respond the way we want them to are always targets for killing among humans. Someone who is brain dead or comatose and who has been abandoned to this state may be a candidate for a quick death to save medical resources. Also, the "inferior," judged by the cost/benefit criteria discussed above, would include the dying. Those who are in the midst of a disease or condition which is shortly to result in death are candidates. A person with a malignant cancer who is judged to be within days of death might be looked upon as a financial burden because of the high medical costs at such times. Quite frankly, the argument goes, "Why not just give them a shot and end their suffering?"

In the long debate over "pulling the plug," it is often stated that such an overdose would appear merciful alongside the wretched death experienced by those who are killed with starvation and thirst. But, isn't it still *killing?* Naturally, a Christian argument is that we shouldn't be killing *any* of them. How much treatment we should give raises many additional questions when dealing with the dying—questions that are not present with people who are merely nonresponsive. We'll discuss their proper treatment elsewhere in the book, but suffice it to say at the moment that this person is alive and is due the same care as any other person.

But, as we saw in other chapters, these people are alive. And, they are people, equal in God's eyes, who should be treated as our neighbors. The list, however, does not end there. The elderly and infirm are included. Also included are people who have chronic illness, irreversible conditions, or who are just too old to defend themselves.

Think about what "chronically ill" means. It means one is not getting any better, but may not necessarily be getting any worse. That may describe a brain dead person, but it also would describe a diabetic or someone with multiple sclerosis, epilepsy, cystic fibrosis, arthritis, or allergies. Those who are handicapped, mentally retarded, or deformed are also at risk. Any of these things could be defined as irreversible as well. Any of them could be very expensive to treat over time. Are we prepared to allow the duty-to-die Lamms of the world to use such broad terminology when it involves killing people?

Neo-Cannibals

With great advances in life-support technology and organ transplantation, the dead today do indeed have much "protein" to offer us—we are the neo-cannibals.
—Nobel Prize-winning virologist,
Carleton Gajdusek

This approving sentiment was expressed by a man who studied a cannibalistic rite among the Fore people of New Guinea, which had been responsible for the spread of a viral condition among them. Absent the viral condition, Gajdusek opined, the Fore people's eating of the brains of their deceased merely "provided a good source of protein for the community."[6]

One of the primary reasons currently used for keeping people alive but simultaneously declaring them brain dead is to benefit the transplant industry. Note the quote at the beginning of this segment referring to the "advances in life-support technology" in relation to what the dead have to offer us.

Organ transplantation is one of those medical arenas that arrived with a flash and a bang and was virtually universally accepted without question. When Christiaan Barnard did the first human-to-human heart transplant in the Groote Schuur Hospital in Pretoria, South Africa, so profound was the astonishment of the world that nary a peep was raised in opposition—with the notable exception of writer and social critic, Malcomb Muggeridge.

When I Give Your Heart, It Will Be Completely

I believe it is a general disregard for life that permits people to think of others as human-parts warehouses. This is particularly evident in heart transplants. The case of Robert Olive, mentioned in another chapter, serves as an example.

Olive was a thief—a person for whom sympathy would be low. The idea that taking his heart would be any kind of crime or immoral act would be ludicrous to some people. They couldn't care less what happened to him.

But, when hearts are stolen from living people with whom we *are* sympathetic, a different tact is taken. The "donor"—and I use that word advisedly since many "donors" have never themselves chosen to donate—will be lionized as a hero who "even in death, gave to others" and who "lives on through others." (Might I note that these are nearly identical to the sayings of the Fore people of New Guinea regarding their dead, whose brains they consume? Gajdusek saw the parallel. But, at least the Fore people didn't, so far as I know, *kill* the object of their next feast.)

However, I don't think it is coincidental that pagan thought in medicine has gained ascendancy at the same time that we have found uses for the bodies of our dead—and, more often, our not-yet-dead. It is true that some people have the donor designations on their driver's licenses checked, but the percentage of U.S. drivers who participate is very small. There are also limitations on whose organs are usable—even if they are freely given. Generally, organs from people beyond their mid-thirties are not used. Organs damaged by trauma or disease are rejected.

So where do all the donations come from? Well, a little-known law, the Uniform Anatomical Gift Act, passed in all fifty states, has already made *you* a donor if your next of kin cannot be reached and your friendly coroner or hospital administrator decides to part you out. You get to give this "gift" whether you want to or not—unless you have a prior written objection. Of course, there is no place on one's driver's license for this. Nor is there any central location to put this objection should you end up in medical hands other than those of your own doctor. The law makes no provision for those who object.

The family of Eleno Ullua Ramirez, a nineteen-year-old Mexican national, found that out in 1989 when Eleno was taken to Hoag Hospital in Costa Mesa, California, after he had been found severely beaten. He carried no identification and police fingerprint identification, when possible, took about forty-eight hours. Within twenty-four hours, the young man was declared brain dead and his heart was extricated and put into Norton Humpheries, a retired doctor.

The family filed suit, but the hospital's response was that it had complied with the law and made a "diligent" search for Eleno's next of kin. "The law is very specific, and we followed the law," said Gail Love, the hospital spokesman. But, she declined to say what this "diligent" search entailed.[7]

Another source of organs is Willard Gaylen's formerly mentioned "neo-morts." Gaylen has suggested that we separate personhood from aliveness by defining the loss of the former as death—essentially cognitive death. In other words, we are no longer a real person if we lose our ability to visibly relate to people and things around us in a coherent fashion. Then Gaylen suggests we maintain the spontaneously breathing human beings for months or years and harvest their parts for transplant and experimental purposes.[8] For these reasons, I have emblazoned "No organs for transplant or experimentation" on both my driver's license and my health care card.

At this time, the American Medical Association's Council on Ethical and Judicial Affairs, the organization's independent policy-making arm, has given approval to taking organ donations from live, anencephalic babies. Anencephalic babies are born without most of their brains, but have a brain stem which controls breathing, heartbeat, the sucking reflex, and other basic functions. They often live only hours, but some live for years.

This pronouncement was the first official approval from the AMA of taking organs from people who are defined by their rules as "alive"—i.e., not brain dead or actually dead. There has been some controversy within the AMA over the decision, but, in the end, it will probably be accepted.

In one case, a Florida couple went to court to have their anencephalic baby girl, Theresa Ann Campo, declared brain dead so they could give out her parts while they were still fresh.[9] The parents and the Thanaphiles who joined them explicitly argued that Theresa must not be allowed to die before the organs were taken lest they become useless. The case, *In re TACP*, was designed to redefine not only anencephalics, but other incompetent patients as "dead." Remember Willard Gaylen's quote in an earlier chapter of the book? "The problem (of euthanasia) is well on its way to being resolved by what must have seemed a relatively simple and ingenious method. As it turned out, the difficult issues of euthanasia could be evaded by redefining death." This was a case to *re*-redefine death. It has worked before, they must have thought, why not try it again? The court eventually denied their request, but that has not stopped the debate and the next court test is likely to be successful.

The point is, Theresa Campo was *not* dead—they admitted as much—but they wanted to use her organs anyway. They wanted to legally declare Theresa dead. Arthur Caplan, director of the Center for Bio-Medical Ethics at the University of Minnesota and a leading "bioethicist," said in 1987, "I don't think these kids are dead, but would I take their organs out? Yes."[10]

And, even if they are not, physicians anxious to use the organs will engage in another kind of legal fiction much like Canadian doctors did with Baby Gabrielle in 1987. Gabrielle, an anencephalic baby, was breathing on her own. As such, she could not be classified as brain dead. This fact alone made her ineligible as an organ donor. So, to avoid the niceties of the law, the medical staff hooked her up to a ventilator (even though she did not need one), declared her brain dead, disconnected the ventilator, cut out her heart, and flew it to California where it was given to another child. No charges were filed or official objections raised.[11]

"I will do what the Aztecs did," said one Canadian physician of his willingness to part out still-living anencephalic babies.[12] As you probably know, the Aztecs sacrificed humans by cutting out their still-beating hearts to sacrifice to the gods.

Regardless of one's beliefs about the morality of transplanting organs, no one could make a case for the transplanting of organs from those who had not voluntarily donated them. Certainly, no one could justify the taking of an organ from a living person which, after its removal, would leave the person dead. Yet, this is often what happens. The brain dead, the comatose, and the anencephalic are more commonly viewed as organ farms than as people. They appear to be a "waste" of good organs.

What's behind the Mask?

Doesn't it seem odd to anyone else that certain members of the medical profession and the media are promoting transplants so heavily? Both spend an inordinate amount of time trying to convince the public to sign up as organ donors—despite the fact that the vast majority of people's organs would be useless for transplant.

What is stranger yet is that medical people and the media lead the Whiner's Club on how expensive and technology-dependent medical care has become. Feeding the elderly is deemed too expensive, while transplants of major organs, costing tens of thousands of dollars, are hailed. This does not even take into consideration the hundreds of dollars per month in costs for anti-rejection medications given to vital organ recipients that they must take for the rest of their lives—or the medical problems that arise from taking these medications. Why do the medical profession and the media seem so driven to involve *everyone* in this business?

It is reminiscent of the abortion debate. Proabortion people don't just want abortion to be a private issue, they want everyone's approval, support, and financial backing. They cannot abide any opposition and *everyone* must help fund this "private decision."

But, the transplant movement misrepresents the concept of "donor" in more ways than one. Besides the Uniform Anatomical Gift Act and the fact that you cannot designate on your driver's license that you *don't* want to be a donor, there are other indicators. Dr. Vivian Tellis, a renal transplant surgeon, is working on a strategy of guilt and pressure on the families of those whom she wishes to be donors. "The family who refuses to donate a dead relative's liver should be told they killed the waiting recipient," she says.[13]

Notice the use of the term *dead* instead of *brain dead* or *comatose*. What would she do with an Orthodox Jewish family who, according to their religion, would object? Impose her own morality? Perhaps she also believes there should be criminal murder charges brought against the family.

Dr. Tellis is not alone in such opinions. Federal law now requires that hospital staff ask family members to donate the organs of their nearly dead relatives. Nor are the motives all that pristine. There is a lot of money in transplantation, as is evidenced by the thriving black market in organs from Third World countries. This has received some coverage in the press. Columnist Gwynne Dyer wrote of the underground organ trade coming out of South America to fulfill the needs of wealthy Americans: "On April 7 [1988], Judge Angel Campos of the Minors' Court in Asuncion, Paraguay, commenting on a case where seven Brazilian baby boys aged between three and six months were rescued from a private home, said, 'The investigations lead us to believe that these babies were going to be butchered in the U.S.' "[14]

Confirmation of similar practices in India comes from the prestigious British medical journal, *Lancet*, saying, "Police in Bangalore city in the southern state of Karnataka claimed to have uncovered a huge interstate kidney transplant racket whereby numerous young men have allegedly been duped of their kidneys unknowingly, or of offers of large sums of money or lucrative jobs promised for their kidneys."[15]

More recently, a British Broadcasting Company program reported that the Chinese government was using executed prisoners as a source of kidney and other organ transplants—both for their own people and for sale to wealthy foreigners at about thirty thousand dollars for a kidney. That same month, the *Eastern Express*, a respected Hong Kong newspaper, reported that there was a thriving business in selling aborted babies to be eaten for purported health and rejuvenation qualities. A female Chinese doctor frankly admitted having eaten "more than 100" of them in the last six months.[16]

Though U.S. law prohibits the selling of the organs themselves, it does not prohibit Americans from buying them elsewhere. Nor does it stop U.S. surgeons and other medical staff from charging fees that "commensurate with the service offered." And, even though the transplant list is supposed to be "first come, first served," there are many instances where wealthy people and prominent politicians seemed to have moved to the head of the line more quickly than ordinary people. Organ transplantation is not a charity operation—and that should tell you something. But, transplant mania has led further and further down the slippery slope.

Grow Your Own Donors

I never thought I'd be pregnant at my age, but when you're faced with the possibility that your child is going to die, you desperately seek, and whatever you need to do, you do it.[17]

—Mary Ayalas, forty-three, who got pregnant to provide a bone-marrow transplant donor for her teen-age daughter who had leukemia

This was a major national news story in 1990. Taking a one-in-four chance that the baby would have compatible bone marrow, this middle-aged woman got pregnant to provide a donor for her teen-age daughter.

If there is legitimacy to organ transplants, it is rooted in the word *consent*. But here, there was not only no consent, there was no consideration of it. In the end, the child's marrow was compatible and was used to save her sister from leukemia. The questions of ethics and morals were never answered. Both children survived, so the "success" was its own overwhelming—and winning—argument.

But, it must have been a foregone conclusion to anyone who observes human nature that with the combination of the transplant craze and the abortion mentality, people would soon be growing their own donors. But, such growing has not stopped at overt "donations" such as organs; it has landed American medicine squarely in the middle of human experimentation and using human bodies to manufacture cures for human ailments.

The Nature of the Cannibal

If cannibalism is strictly defined as the eating of human flesh, the Fore people of New Guinea and the late convicted murderer Jeffery Dahmer would be the only kinds of people who would qualify. But, I think cannibalism goes deeper than that. For a better definition, we need to look at why cannibalism took place.

Historically, there have been a number of justifications for cannibalism given by the societies that practiced it. One would be just plain survival—the need for food. Another involves religious ideas. The ancient Aztecs used to rip the hearts out of their tens of thousands of sacrificial victims, usually captives from war, and offer the hearts to the sun god in order to keep it lit. The remainder of the body was given to the warrior who captured the man to be shared in a feast with his family. The idea was to acquire the strength of the warrior's enemy for himself and his family. Because warriors tended to respect their opponents, the main "guest" at this feast was seen to be living on in the man who defeated him. Other societies, such as the Fore, ate those who died naturally within their tribe as a way for those people to find "continued existence." Eating your friends or enemies was often done in association with religious rites whose purpose was attaining the blessings of prosperity and health for the tribe and all its members. Partaking of the "meal" insured these blessings of the gods.

The Klonds of India actually raised a tribe of people like cattle, the Meriahs, for the exclusive purpose of human sacrifice.

The reason I bring up human sacrifice as part of this discussion is because of the alignment of effects and purpose with cannibalism. Both 1) kill innocent people, and 2) use their bodies to secure some "good" for others. In the normal sense of the term *human sacrifice*, the body of the person is offered for a god to "consume" on behalf of the tribe. The "consumption" may not be done by the individuals of the tribe, but the tribe has vicariously consumed both the life and the body of the sacrifice victim for their own good. To me, the consumption (through

whatever means) of a human body for purposes of
survival defines cannibalism. The fact that similar
justifications are offered for human organ transplantation and experimentation only serves to seal
the nature of what we are doing.

But, if organ transplantation and human experimentation cannot be strictly defined as cannibalism in the minds of some, it might be more
easily seen as human sacrifice. Either practice leaves
the victim just as dead. We should look at some of
our current medical practices with this reasoning in
mind. The example above of the woman who became pregnant in order to supply a bone-marrow
donor for her older child has a remarkably similar
ring to the Klonds' raising the Meriahs for the
purposes of sacrifice.

For millennia, cannibalism has had medicinal
uses in some cultures. "The most remarkable examples of the practice occur in China. Among the
poor it is not uncommon for a member of the family to cut off a piece of flesh from arm or leg, which
is cooked and given to the sick relative."[18]

The example of the woman having a child for
the purposes of a bone-marrow transplant has no-
ticeable similarities and was, at the time, an isolated
case. But, other similar cases have been reported
since. On several occasions, people have planned to
get pregnant in order to deliberately obtain a third-
trimester abortion and salvage the organs for a family member. But, even these might be considered
isolated if it were not for the burgeoning industry
of fetal experimentation and harvesting. The gruesome march of technological death goes on—as we
shall see.

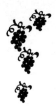

Chapter Seven

Lampshades, Anyone?

Wir haben nichts davon gewusst [We didn't know].[1]
—Villagers near the Nazi death camps

People in the prolife movement are familiar with incidents where unborn babies were used for artwork, earrings, paperweights, and other profane things. There are also cosmetics which use collagen from aborted babies, though these are rare (and very expensive). These chilling tales remind us of the infamous Nazi lampshades that were made from human skin. However, a much deeper evil is being perpetrated—human experimentation.

The lampshades may have been an anomaly, but the Nazis were the ultimate recyclers, and the hair of their victims was baled and sent off to be made into fabric for liners in army uniforms, bones were pulverized for fertilizer or used to "gravel" icy roads, fat was boiled and made into soap, and the gold was plucked from the corpses' teeth. They used everything but the screams of their victims.

But, also in the Nazi death camps, many experiments took place on living human beings. People were injected with foreign substances. Newborns were tortured to death to study the reactions of their mothers to seeing their own children in pain. Children had their eyes injected with blue dye to see if they could be converted to Aryans. Men were immersed in freezing water to see if certain drugs would slow hypothermia. The list was endless. So was the supply of guinea pigs.

The Nuremberg War Crimes Trials sorted all this out. Doctors were not allowed to escape with flimsy excuses. A whole new set of guidelines—the Nuremberg Code—was adopted. For decades, the scientific data from those experiments was considered anathema by the medical profession steeped in Christian medical ethics. In more recent times, that barrier has been broken and the results of those tests are being taken seriously. The argument has been made that there might be some beneficial information contained in the records of this barbarity. Pragmatic concerns have overridden moral concerns and the data has begun to be searched for useful information.

One might not be so concerned with this if it were not evident that some medical science practitioners of our day are altogether too prepared to conduct similar experiments themselves. Today, it is not Jews and other concentration camp inmates who are the subjects, but other kinds of "inferior" people that the Thanaphiles are trying to kill. In many cases, these "inferior" people fit the description of the other victims of the Nazis—the handicapped, mentally retarded, and others killed in the Reich's euthanasia program.

In 1988, Dr. Alain Milhaud of Amiens, France, had his license to practice medicine suspended by the health minister for performing an experiment on Pacal Louette, twenty-four, a comatose patient. The patient died. Milhaud was once (in 1985) charged with experimenting on another comatose man, but the investigation did not prove a direct connection between the death of that patient and the unauthorized experiment. At the time of the first experiment, the good doctor called the comatose "almost perfect models who constitute intermediaries between animal and man."[2] Only the Lord knows how many experiments he did for which he did not get caught. Not commented upon in this story is the fact that this charming doctor was never cited for the unauthorized experimentation, but only the possibility that the experiment caused the death.

Currently, the craze is experimenting on unborn babies—often obtained from abortions. Much has been made of this in the newspapers, but one central lie prevails—that fetal experiments have been prohibited by law. The truth is that the only thing prohibited by law was *federal funding* of the experiments. While such things as earrings, paperweights, and "art" using human fetuses may be the exception, it does not lessen the horror of the common, experimental uses to which these children are put.

Dark Cures

The bodies of aborted infants are currently being used in experimental cures for adult diseases. Nigel Davies, in his aforementioned book, noted that this was also a common practice among tribes practicing human sacrifice and cannibalism. The difference is that today's "cures" are purported to be scientific. What is not different is the morality of using these children's bodies for medicine—even if it is effective.

Many of us have read about pancreatic cells being implanted into diabetics so that they can produce their own insulin. A recent U.S. trial of the Russian technique showed "marked improvement" for the diabetics, but death for the babies.[3] These cells come almost exclusively from unborn babies. It is also well known that there is ongoing work with fetal brain cells being injected into people with Parkinson's disease to help stop the brain degeneration. The fetal cells, it is said, are still in a growth mode and are adaptable enough to integrate into the brain of the patient. But, abortion has a way of grinding up and destroying babies to the point where their tissue becomes useless for transplant, so new methods have been developed.

One of the most grisly modern revelations was of an abortion technique perfectly suited to harvesting tissue and organs from aborted babies. Abortionist Martin Haskell of Cincinnati, Ohio, delivered a paper to the 1992 National Abortion Federation Risk Management Seminar. He called the procedure, specifically designed for late second and for third-trimester babies, dilation and extraction or D&X. It consists of dilating the cervix, reaching inside the womb with forceps, grasping the unanesthetized child's leg and drawing it down out of the womb causing a breech, or feet-first, partial delivery. The head, which, in this procedure, is too large to fit through the cervix, is still inside the mother, so the abortionist creates a wound at the base of the skull with scissors. A suction catheter is inserted into the wound and the brain tissue is suctioned out. This collapses the skull for easy removal. The touted advantage to this procedure is that it both insures the death of the child and isn't as messy as the D&E (dilation and evacuation) where the child is dismembered by the forceps and removed in pieces. Another "advantage" is that the various organs and tissues, so versatile for transplant, are preserved intact.[4]

Nonconsenting Adults

There are great advantages to testing medical procedures on human subjects, but there are also specific rules that apply to doing so. The first rule is consent—*informed* consent. The second is that there must be some potential benefit for the subject of the test. Tests that do not offer some hope of benefit are called "non-therapeutic." Nazi doctors were condemned to their deaths for experimenting on prisoners, even on their remains after they died, without informed consent. The Nuremberg Tribunal, who condemned them, would not accept the rationale that the prisoners were going to die anyway.

Even those who only received body parts for experiments from already-dead prisoners were judged guilty. The Nuremberg Code said that "the voluntary consent of the human subject is absolutely essential. . . . The duty and responsibility for ascertaining the quality of the consent rests upon each individual who initiates . . . the experiment."[5] The Code also forbids withholding treatment or care for "scientific" reasons barring an informed consent that one might be a part of a "control group receiving a placebo." In other words, no scientific gain is to be worth the involuntary suffering of others.

But, the horror of those experiments did not sink into the American consciousness as far as one would have hoped. In 1972 it became known that the U.S. Public Health Service had allowed six hundred nonconsenting, black, Tuskeegee, Alabama, men to suffer untreated from syphilis for twenty years in order to ascertain the course of the disease. These men had given no informed consent, and the experiment was nontherapeutic. One would think that the shocking discovery of this appalling "study" would have reinforced all the pronouncements of the Nuremberg Code, but not so.

The burden of becoming experimental fodder has merely shifted to a new group of nonhumans. Much of the 1972 shock over the Tuskeegee experiment was related to the new sensitivity about black people being what they had been all along—real people. So, medical science had to find a suitable replacement for black men, and found it one year later when the U.S. Supreme Court declared unborn babies to be nonpersons. The decision did not address fetal experimentation, but the loophole was large enough to drive a truckload of nontherapeutic scalpels through—and the Thanaphiles did not hesitate.

Suzanne Rini, a journalist, author of *Beyond Abortion: A Chronicle of Fetal Experimentation*, and arguably the nation's foremost expert on the issue of fetal experimentation, told me in a radio interview that she has come to the conclusion that the legalization of abortion came about because of the pressure from the fetal experimentation and tissue transplant industries, not, as some believe, the other way around.

Since it would be impossible to gain the informed consent of an unborn baby, the medical profession has opted for consent of the mother. This is obtained at abortion facilities by including language about "tissue disposal" in the consent form that is shoved under every abortion-bound mother's nose at the clinic before her child is killed. These forms are almost never read and the "tissue disposal" language could hardly be described as giving "informed" consent that her child may become someone's guinea pig.

Consent of the parent, under other circumstances, may be sufficient for trying an experimental procedure on a child, but this is where the hope of success comes in. In normal experimental procedures on children, there is at least a chance that the child himself will benefit from the attempt. With aborted children, there is no such hope. All of the procedures either require or cause their deaths.

Lab Rats

I have often affectionately called my children, when they were young, and now my grandchildren, "rug rats," without ever imagining that they should be treated as actual rats. But, the scientist interested in fetal experimentation thinks differently. It is "lab rats" he seeks—or better yet, human tissue. There are four groups of unborn infants used in experimentation:

1) The live, in-utero fetus. Scientists test drugs, vaccines, prenatal diagnostic techniques (search-and-

destroy) such as chorionic villi sampling, and other things on children who are still alive in their mother's wombs but are slated for abortion. After the abortion, the child's body is studied for the effects of the experimental drug or procedure.

2) The living, viable (able to survive outside the womb), ex-utero fetus. Similar testing can be done on this aborted child—essentially a premature infant brought to delivery purposely. Organs can also be harvested from them if the tests do not damage the organ tissues. Experiments done on these infants are not paid for through tax funds, but there is no bar to privately funded research of this kind.

3) The "pre-viable" (unable to survive outside the womb) fetus, ex- or in-utero. This child is defined in federal regulations as one who has been or is about to be aborted—though possibly still living. If they have not already been killed, they always have vital signs and, as such, are alive.

4) The dead fetus. In this case, clinically dead, the child is simply used as parts for experimentation or transplant.[6]

In every case, the Nuremberg Code is violated. The children have become little more than soulless lab rats. Even convicted serial murderers have more protection.

What They Do in the Dark

As we have said, the earrings and paperweights are an anomaly, but the experimentation is common and even more sickening. From Rini's book, we learn of many such experiments. In 1975 it was revealed in an article called "The Dutch Famine," that researchers had starved pregnant women prior to their abortions to study the effects of malnutrition on developing babies. This was conducted when federal funding for fetal experimentation was forbidden and a special commission was meeting to determine the ethics of such ventures. But, private funds were available and the meeting of the commission did not slow the researchers' work. This was not the only such experiment conducted.

In Helsinki, Finland, a group of live-born aborted babies had their heads severed from their bodies and placed in a solution to see how long the brains could be kept alive. U.S. taxpayer dollars were involved, as was funding from March of Dimes.[7]

The Catholic University of Notre Dame authorized a cell-culture experiment from the cerebrum of a twenty-week-old diseased baby who had been aborted by use of Prostaglandin E;[8] prostaglandin abortions are notorious for producing live births, making them a favorite technique for those seeking experimental subjects. Since live responses are desired by these researchers, these babies are very likely to have been born alive and vivisected.

No animal studies preceded the fetal research where living babies of seven months gestation were aborted and hooked up to artificial placentas and immersed in an oxygenated solution. An Ohio medical research company tested brain, heart, and other organs as part of a pesticide research contract with the U.S. Environmental Protection Agency. In both 1973 and 1976, infants aborted alive were sliced open and had their sex organs and adrenal glands removed for experimentation.

But, one of the most common uses of fetal tissue is to develop "cell lines" for culturing diseases for further study or vaccines to stop disease. The child's cells, which are living and very versatile, are placed in a solution that allows them to continue living and growing new cells. These cells are then infected with a disease the researchers wish to study or with a weakened strain of a disease for which they wish to have vaccines. The military and other government agencies—and even cosmetic manufacturers—have benefited from this "cell line" research.[9] In fact, this line of inquiry has proven to be a boon for the medical profession. The fact that the medicines developed from these murder victims have been effective has drowned out the moral questions raised by these procedures. But remember, the continuously multiplying cells are a still-living part of that child who was murdered and used as a medicine for others.

In one case in England, it became known that a vaccine had been cultured in this way. Catholics and Moslems were in an uproar and refused to allow their children to be inoculated with a vaccine derived from a murder victim.[10] They rightly realized that to *knowingly* participate would make them complicit in the murder of the child from whom the cell line was stolen. How many times have you been injected with the cells of a murder victim as part of a treatment or vaccine? That may be hard to tell, as most vaccines come from chicken embryos. But, if you or your children have participated in the common vaccinations, like rubella, given in this country, it is possible that you or they have been unwitting beneficiaries of this morally bankrupt form of research.

Who Pays?

The simple answer to that question is: You do. If you have ever contributed to the March of Dimes, the Muscular Dystrophy Association, or the American Paralysis Association, your money may have gone to these gruesome experiments. Rini's research revealed that all of these organizations have funded fetal experimentation. March of Dimes was primarily responsible for the search-and-destroy techniques of amniocentesis and chorionic villi sampling (CVS) which were developed through live fetal research. Not only did the development of amniocentesis and CVS cost the lives of untold numbers of unborn children, it also results in the accidental deaths of about 2–3 percent of the children on whom it is used.[11] Amniocentesis is exclusively used to find and abort "defective" infants. None of the medical problems which amniocentesis can detect can be corrected in the womb, so there can be no other purpose for the test than to pressure the mother into aborting a "defective" child.

Foundations also loom large in fetal research money. By far the largest and most consistent supporter of eugenic policies and practices is the Rockefeller Foundation. But money also has flowed from the Ford Foundation and McDonald's Kroc Medical Foundation among others.[12]

Many recall the sense of victory when Presidents Reagan and Bush each vetoed fetal experimentation funding bills. Most people misunderstood the bills as being laws prohibiting fetal experimentation itself, but they represented funding only. Some states have laws prohibiting the experimentation itself, but they are largely ignored and unenforced.

Suzanne Rini says,

> Under current [1988] regulations, one may
> do anything except a procedure that stops
> the heart. But it is quite possible to remove
> vital organs, even the heart, without stop-
> ping the heart *directly*. Researchers themselves
> have proven that. . . . The U.S. regulations
> do not state that a previable fetus must be
> void of heartbeat before being dissected or
> experimented on. (emphasis added)[13]

But, in 1993, President Bill Clinton, as a pur-
poseful slap in the face to prolife America, chose
the twentieth anniversary of the *Roe vs. Wade* abortion decision and the day that more than one hundred thousand prolifers marched in memorial of the
thirty-two million dead babies, to sign five execu-
tive orders undoing all the prolife gains of the last
decade—including lifting the ban on federal funding for fetal experimentation. So, even if your money
never went to any of the foundations or organizations which have funded the fetal research, you have
now, through your tax dollars, become a participant. U.S. government funders include National In-
stitute of Child Health and Development under the
Department of Health and Human Services, the
Food and Drug Administration, the Environmental
Protection Agency, the U.S. Agency for International Development, and the U.S. military.[14]

"Rational" Motives

*I accepted those brains, of course: where they came
from and how they came to me was really none of my
business.*

—A German physician during
the Nuremberg trials

These could almost be the words of one of the fetal experimenters today. In fact, it chillingly mirrors the statement of a female Chinese doctor who was one of those interviewed about eating aborted babies that was mentioned in the last chapter. She was the one who admitted to having eaten more than one hundred in the previous six months. She said, "They are wasted if we don't eat them. The women who receive abortions here don't want the fetuses."[15] The rationalization did not work for the Nazis, and it shouldn't work now. Remember the Nuremberg Code says that the responsibility for gaining and verifying consent lies with the experimenter.

In Germany, there was no use getting consent from a legal nonperson—a Jew, for instance. So, today in America, the idea of getting consent from the unborn seems just as useless. To today's researcher it would seem as foolish as it would have been for the German physician to get consent from the *Juden* in 1930s Germany. We are all blinded to our own times by cultural myopia. But, there is more than one rationale for what Suzanne Rini calls "Frankenstein science."

Joseph Fletcher, who seems to pop up every time someone needs to explain why it is all right to kill somebody, has explained that, considering the brutality of abortion procedures, the experiments are quite tame. He says that we may use these children so long as they are unwanted—that it is "wantedness" which would give the children enough value to make the experiments unethical.

Fletcher, of course, ignores the many brutal experiments that have been done on the unborn. And, he also relies upon the fallacy that a lesser evil is justified by its avoidance of a greater evil. We won't rob them and kill them, we'll just rob them.

Proverbs 12:10 tells us that even the kindness of the wicked is cruel. Other people speak of the general good of mankind brought about with the fetal experiments. The development of the rubella vaccine from testing on fetal tissue lines is often mentioned. But, others say that such tests could easily have been replicated on animal tissue. A number of ethicists have noted that as much work as possible should be done on animals before the beginning of human testing. The fact is, however, that many of the fetal experiments done are never preceded by animal tests. This is probably due to the easy access and unrestricted use allowed with human fetal tissue as opposed to animals. The animal rights movement has been so successful in its efforts that animal testing is severely limited and very expensive due to the regulations.

The perversity of animal versus human rights could not have been more obvious than in a 1995 interview with Dr. Mike McCune, who, as a postdoctoral fellow at Stanford University, successfully transplanted components of the immune systems of unborn children into mice—creating what he called Mouse Man or SCID-hu (Severe Combined ImmunoDeficiency-human mouse) for his studies of AIDS and HIV. Not a word was breathed in the article about the morality of using human being parts for the experiments or where those parts came from, but the interviewer was sure to ask about the animal rights questions.

What do animal rights groups think of your research? Have there been any face-to-face confrontations? If it isn't already evident, would you like to justify using animals in your research for any of the readers who might categorize themselves as animal rights advocates?

We've been very cognizant that animal research is something you have to be careful about. In the early days, we called the SCID-hu mouse the Mouse Man, but the animal rights group thought this was overly pejorative—mostly against the mouse.

Most of the activity of animal rights groups is rightfully directed, I think, at ill-conceived experiments that inflict unnecessary pain on animals. We have tried, when constructing the SCID-hu, to steer clear of those problems. We've put a great deal of effort into the design of our protocols to ensure that they can answer the questions in a meaningful way and that they are humane. Overlaying this is the goal: we are using animals to help us make decisions about which drugs to take into the clinic. If we don't have those decisions made for us in the animal model, we'll be using other animals, namely humans, to make the same decision.[16]

When I read this, the prolifer in me screams out, "What about the babies? You are *already* using humans—the babies!" But, as things stand, there are currently many regulations on using animal subjects. There are no *de facto* regulations which cause any such problem with unborn babies as test sub-

jects. They have no lobby, and, because of the prevalent proabortion attitude, any regulations that do
exist will likely be ignored.

Today many researchers say that new computer
models can often give as accurate an answer to our
questions as any live tissue research. But, even if
technology could not simulate live tissue research,
experiments on nonconsenting, defenseless children
who have no chance of benefiting from how their
bodies are used and abused could not possibly fit
any model of Christian morality or ethics.

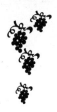

Chapter Eight

Thanaphiles in Thanatasia

Death is a very good way to cut expenses.
—Woody Allen

Death has become the solution to many of our problems. If people are too old, too sick, or just too much trouble, our solution is to kill them outright or "allow them to die." It saves money. Maybe, they slyly hint, if we let doctors do it, the killing will seem more sanctified somehow. Viktor Brack, a Nazi doctor and head of the Third Reich Chancellery's Euthanasia Department II, claimed the same thing when he said, "The syringe belongs in the hand of the physician."[1]

During the campaign for physician-assisted suicide in the state of Oregon, this was one of the prime arguments. If doctors did it, it wouldn't be corrupted. Christians, who understand the natural corruption of man, should know otherwise. In a Bioethics symposium held at the time, Dr. John M. Dolan of the University of Minnesota said: "To say, 'We can't give this power to kill to just anybody— let's give it to doctors because they've proven over thousands of years that they protect life' is like saying, 'We can't trust just anybody to drown people, let's let the lifeguards do it.' "

The point is well made. After thousands of years of proving that, unlike ancient pagan medicine men, physicians, in general, could be trusted with your life, the Thanaphiles want to destroy that trust, which took twenty-four hundred years to build.

Thus, the euthanasia movement hopes to sanitize killing. But, Dr. Dolan argues that, by definition, a physician is one who protects life and heals and that "physician-assisted suicide" is a contradiction in terms.

Thanaphiles, while currently arguing for the physician to assist in euthanasia, have plans to broaden the scope.

Fables of "Good" Death

Euthanasia—in the Greek, "good death"—originally meant that a person died, relatively pain-free, surrounded by family and with all of his household in order. Now, it is always associated with killing people the way one does an injured horse or dog.

But, euthanasia is described in many categories which are designed, in part, to bring confusion to the average person. The first of these is called "passive" euthanasia. The vision promoted of passive euthanasia is that of allowing someone to die as opposed to keeping them alive with machines. In other words, the person is not directly killed by any action taken by another. Rather, they die because of the *inaction* of another. An example would be when they stop giving an elderly person antibiotics and

allow the next infection—pneumonia, for instance—
to kill them.

The difficulty here arises in the difference between the promoted image of passive euthanasia
and the reality of the practice. Is the inaction bringing about a death from the disease or condition or
is the person dying from something that is treatable
when treatment has been refused? This is the question that must be answered.

Another example of so-called passive euthanasia is the withholding of food and water or antibiotics from a brain dead or comatose person. Was
the person dying of a condition other than their
brain dead or comatose state? Or were they just
elderly? Was it that condition which killed him or
the lack of food and water or treatment for a simple
infection? If there was no other fatal condition which
killed him, there was nothing passive about this
euthanasia. Sure, the person was not given a lethal
injection, but the removal of ordinary care and treatment was *intended* to kill. It is another matter if a
person is on the verge of death and antibiotics are
not administered because they would have no real
hope of lengthening life or bringing comfort to the
dying person. But, when a person dies from something other than a fatal condition because of the
deliberate inaction of the medical staff, and that
inaction is *intended* to bring about death, it is nothing short of killing.

Nor is it "allowing to die" when another vital
need, such as air is withheld. If a person needs
assistance to breathe, via ventilator, it is no different than their needing to be spoon-fed. Removal of

that aid (barring the person's suffering fatal bodily failures elsewhere), is intended to kill. In most cases, this is what is happening in the cases labeled passive euthanasia.

"Active" euthanasia is the case everyone always pictures with a doctor giving a lethal injection to a patient and having the patient fall peacefully into the hands of death. Most Christians recognize this as pure murder. However, after having been presented with all the other kinds of killing—by starvation and so forth—the lethal injection seems almost compassionate. But, one should not allow the emotional issue to cloud the facts: both are the intentional killing of innocent people, nothing less! The difference is merely the difference between a sin of omission or commission. Either way, the patient is murdered.

Volunteers

One aspect of euthanasia that seems to confuse people is whether or not it is voluntary. In order to be voluntary, the decision must come from a person who is awake, aware, and competent. In such a case, it is nothing more than secondhand suicide—assisted suicide.

The point is not who assists the person, but the simple fact of suicide. Suicide means that the last act you will commit on earth is murder. If you get someone—doctor or not—to assist you, you have an accomplice to murder who is just as culpable before God as you are.

While God may be able to sort out who committed suicide because of true mental defect, and is therefore not accountable for the act, we rarely know that. The Christian Church has historically treated suicide as a form of murder and, so grave was the sin, refused any Christian burial to suicides.

While suicide may be a one-time situation for the victim, euthanasia, for its accomplices, is evidently addictive. In the Netherlands, for example, euthanasia is not truly legal, but is practiced openly. Doctors are allowed to kill so long as certain guidelines are followed. Whatever convinced them that mere guidelines would be followed where they had failed to enforce actual laws, I'll never know. Since that time, however, the Netherlands has become a model for the Thanaphiles. But, it is not the wonderful paradise of choice that they make it out to be. A Dutch government report in 1990 revealed that there had been more than 11,000 *reported* euthanasias that year. Out of the total, 5,941—*more than half*—had been involuntary. And, these were only the physicians who would *admit* to nonvoluntary euthanasia!

Now, to understand the significance of this, remember that euthanasia is *illegal* there but that their supreme court has ruled that it should not be prosecuted if certain guidelines are followed. The very first guideline is that the patient's request must be voluntary! The death ethic apparently has such a blinding hold on that nation that the doctors are not even afraid to tell the government that they not only disobeyed the law, but they disobeyed the guideline of voluntariness. And, nothing was done to the doctors for killing patients who had not asked for death.

What is happening now is that there has come a presumption of death, as opposed to the presumption of life discussed in an earlier chapter. People who do not respond the way we want them to are presumed to be dead. Worse yet, people who don't (and can't) volunteer to die are presumed to want to die. Those who expressly have stated that they don't want to die, are being presumed to be incompetent to make such decisions—and are being killed anyway. Death never says, "Enough!"

Living Wills and Living Won'ts

Helga Wanglie didn't want to die—in fact, she was "biologically tenacious." So great was her desire to live all the life God gave her that she had explicitly stated on many occasions that she wanted "everything" done to keep her alive in the event of her being unable to communicate. Her faith, she had said to her husband, Oliver, was that when God wanted her dead, she would die, but that she intended to live every minute until that time. If there had been a legal document available which would have been the opposite of a living will, she would have signed it. As it was, she had only her husband to witness her firm conviction. Her husband of fifty-four years honored that request when, elderly and severely brain damaged, Helga was placed in Hennepin County Medical Center in Minneapolis, Minnesota, in May of 1990.

But, this expressed desire was not pleasing to the hospital staff, who wanted to unplug Helga's ventilator in spite of her husband's refusal to give permission. So, the hospital took the case to court to try to force the death of Helga Wanglie. Fortunately, the judge who heard the case was unconvinced by the "health care providers" and, on 1 July 1991, granted Oliver Wanglie the sole right to make medical decisions for his wife.[2] She died of natural causes shortly after the ruling.

Why is it that there are living wills, but no living won'ts? Why is it that hospitals like Hennepin County Medical Center in Minnesota and Sacred Heart Hospital in Spokane, Washington (where they tried to kill Baby Ryan Nguyen) insist on death in spite of the wishes of the patient or their next-of-kin? Why would they talk about patient choice and go to court to violate it?

I think the answers are insidious. Some medical staff tend to view themselves as gods—as a cut above others, if only in making medical decisions. This pride is easily manipulated by the spiritual forces behind the pagan death ethic. There needs to be no arcane, back-room conspiracy where there is a shared spirit of paganism. Once death is seen as a solution to social (not to mention financial) problems, the tendency to use it more and more becomes addictive. After years of hyping the distant possibility that everyone would die writhing in pain hooked up to countless machines, the Thanaphiles convinced most states to pass living will laws. These laws provided a legal instrument for frightened people to sign which would "allow you to provide basic direction about decision making in the event of a terminal condition." This is incredible in an age where we have more and better drugs for relieving pain than at any other time in human history.

But, the forms, while appearing to give the person autonomy, are nearly worthless. None are specific enough to cover the contingencies which will probably arise during such a crisis. Worse, the language is usually so vague that a doctor could deny insulin to a diabetic (diabetes is an incurable disease) or to a comatose patient under the guise of stopping "heroic" medical efforts and treatment. Or, he could simply starve the patient to death. As we have noted, many conditions can be called incurable and even terminal, though maybe not immediately so. Living wills are replete with such terms.

Living wills are a trap. Conscientious doctors say that they are vague and so they cannot stop treatments or care which would result in death, while other doctors use that very vagueness to end the lives of people with curable maladies.

The purpose of the living will—or advance directive—is to free someone other than yourself to make those decisions in a pinch. That someone else will be the medical staff who wheel you in. They will interpret the document according to their own bent. Signing a living will can be tantamount to telling them that you don't want to have any serious attempt made to save your life. The Thanaphiles would have you believe that it is actually *your* wishes that are being followed, but remember Helga Wanglie. Her wishes were not respected. She was one of the few fortunate enough to have a judge who didn't buy the Thanaphile lie. Nancy Ellen Jobes, Claire Conroy, Christine Bussalachi, and Nancy Cruzan all were not so fortunate. They didn't have living wills, but the courts ruled that they would have wanted one and signed their death warrants. And, if the doctor misrepresents or misunderstands what you wanted, you will not survive to challenge his judgment.

I used to think it would be possible to write a living will that would adequately cover the contingencies, but I no longer believe it is possible to succeed in that. A friend of mine attended a Human Life International White Rose Conference on euthanasia in Santa Clara, California, in 1991, where one medical ethicist, Monsignor William Smitty opposed living wills and proposed that the only medical directive he would sign would, in the event of his terminal illness, instruct his family and friends to prop him up on a beach in Hawaii and "give me Piña Coladas until I die of natural causes."

Even some Christians have been lulled by the siren song of death. They have come up with a variant of the living will called the Christian Affirmation of Life, which merely puts a spiritual face on all the greasy language used to kill the sick instead of trying to heal them. The same ambiguities exist in the Christian version as in the secular one. And remember, the living will is merely a wedge to widen the euthanasia door. Derek Humphery, euthanasia enthusiast and founder of the Hemlock Society, a proeuthanasia group, said in a 1989 interview, "We have to go stage by stage, with the living will, with the power of attorney, with the withdrawal of this; we have to go stage by stage. Your side would call this the 'slippery slope.'"

I would advise, in the words of Paul Byrne, physician, neonatologist, and expert on brain death and euthanasia:

1) Do not sign a living will or any of its variants, such as the Christian Affirmation of Life. If you have signed one, rescind it in writing immediately and be sure to destroy *every* copy.

2) Do not sign any advance directive that would deny you treatment on the basis of such vague and life-endangering language as:
* artificial means
* benefit
* care appropriate to my condition
* incurable condition, irreversible coma
* inevitable and imminent death
* natural death, prolonging dying.

3) Do not sign any advance directive that would deny you:
* life-sustaining or life-prolonging procedures
* heroic measures
* futile treatment.[3]

All of the terms above—artificial, incurable, imminent, futile, and the like—are simply too vague to interpret properly.

So, write your own statement that you want *all* possible care and treatment. Period. Just such a form, the Life Support Directive, is available through Citizens United Resisting Euthanasia.[4] Sign one before you are in the position where you can be declared incompetent to do so by some court as happened to Marjorie Nighbert. If you want to refuse specific kinds of care after that, you are still free to do so. I have considered calling these living won'ts, or Wanglie wills in honor of Helga, the woman discussed at the start of this chapter portion.

No Substitutions

The right of an adult who, like Claire Conroy, was once competent, to determine the course of her medical treatment remains intact even when she is no longer able to assert that right or to appreciate its effectuation.
                    —New Jersey Supreme Court

Read that quote again—carefully. Can you see what that means? It says that Claire Conroy can decide to starve herself to death even though she cannot now make that decision for herself. She can choose to die even if she's incapable of choosing it for herself. The concept is called "substituted judgment" and it means that once you are declared incompetent, someone else may substitute their own judgment for yours (for your own good, of course). An Arizona court ruled in the case of Mildred Rasmussen that a person may choose to die even if her illness is not terminal and even if a guardian does the deciding for her.

Many states are encouraging people to pick their own substitute with what is called a "durable power of attorney," as mentioned in the Derek Humphery quote earlier. The danger in doing this is that no one knows how this person would react to the pressure from medical staff clamoring for transplant material or giving you the "compassionate" treatment. With a firm statement in hand that you want to be treated as alive as long as you are alive, a relative or friend is a good thing to have to guard your life against overly anxious social engineers

worried about where the money for your hospital
bed is going to come from.

DNR

When someone's heart stops, medical staff swing
into action to perform cardiopulmonary resuscitation (CPR)—at least, they used to. Today, the ad-
ministering of CPR is dependent on which patient
you are talking about. Those who are on the very
edge of death from another disease and, as often,
those who have chronic, deteriorating conditions
are often placed on the DNR list—the do not re-
suscitate list.

In the case of the cancer victim whose life is
going to end within hours or days, one can understand why the medical staff would not want to res-
urrect a patient for just a few more hours of suffering. But, the person with the chronic heart condition might live for years if resuscitated. The DNR
status can be requested by the patient, but more
often, it is placed there by medical staff without the
patient's permission if the staff believe such care is
inappropriate.

According to Earl Appleby, Jr., of Citizens
United Resisting Euthanasia (CURE), several ver-
sions of DNR have surfaced in hospitals across the
country—many of which are apparently intended to
be surreptitious. In one case, a Queens, New York
hospital placed a stick-on purple dot on the charts
of those upon whom a DNR order had been placed.
The dots were removed after the patients' deaths to
cover up the DNR designation. Other places passed
the DNR from shift to shift by word of mouth or

penciled it in on the nursing card index where it could be erased after the patient's demise.

Often the DNR will be called a "No Code" or "No Code Blue." In some places, there was in place a "Slow Code" which Appleby quotes the *Ontario Medical Review* as referring to "start CPR, but only after we have coffee."[5] A friend, who once worked in Physicians and Surgeons Hospital in Portland, Oregon, says that when she worked there, the phrase used was, "Walk slowly, don't run."

Arcane symbols are sometimes used or, the Thanaphile favorite, euphemisms such as "compassionate care only." This last means that only ordinary care items like food, water, and pain control are offered. I suppose that this may be an improvement over those who want to withdraw food and water, but the intent in both cases is a dead patient.

A "Light Code Blue" was adopted in some places to let the staff perform "token activity," according to the New York Task Force on Life and Law, to make it *appear* the patient was being worked on "for the benefit of the family," but having the same end result as the DNR—namely, death.[6]

But, some institutions are seeking what they are describing as voluntary DNRs. A friend of mine, Lisa, called me one night a few years ago telling me of an elderly, low-income man, Daniel, who was being placed in a nursing home down the street from us. She was frantic. They were just trying to kill him, she claimed. Sure enough, when I went with her to this place, they were "requiring" him to sign a DNR before admitting him. Since his care was government funded, he had little choice of places to go, and his two strokes had not left him in much of a condition to argue with them. I have since found out that this has become standard procedure in many nursing homes—particularly government-owned facilities or those receiving government-paid patients. So much for the prodeath camp's cries for choice.

"Imminent" Death

There is a fiction that doctors and other medical staff are able to predict approximately when death will occur. This becomes less accurate as the prediction is made over a greater length of time. A prediction of hours is more likely to be close than one measured in months. Yet this predictability forms the basis of many euthanasia arguments, including the Oregon law passed in 1994 which allows physician-assisted suicide. But, even Thanaphiles will admit that this proffered prognosticating power of medical people is a myth. Thousands of people survive their doctors' direst predictions.

"Imminent" may be properly used of us all in the context of certainty rather than immediacy. We are all certain to die. But, the further away one tries to predict death, the less likely he is to be correct. One may, with much greater confidence, predict a death within hours or a few days of certain advanced cases, but when predicting death within six months, the odds against accuracy rise exponentially.

When Dr. Peter Goodwin, an ardent supporter of Oregon's euthanasia law, was asked, "Can a doctor tell if a person has less than six months to live?"

he answered, "Absolutely not." This kind of answer has been nearly universal by Thanaphiles.

So, why are they promoting these proeuthanasia laws for those "within six months of death" if this cannot be known? Quite simply they are just trying to open the door wider to the killing. As soon as those laws are in place, these same people will say that the six-month period is arbitrary and the whole thing of timing should be left solely to the doctor's discretion and the patient's choice. Then we will have many deaths like Jack Kevorkian's first killing, Janet Adkins, who was years away from death from Alzheimer's disease.

Soon, as is done in the Netherlands and as Kevorkian has done on at least one occasion, there will be assistance in the deaths of those who are merely depressed. The only thing imminent is that the next phase of killing is upon us.

Futility

The most recent development in the Thanaphiles' use of language is "futile treatment." They will make the claim that certain life-saving or life-sustaining treatment would be futile in certain cases. This, however, does not mean it would not be *effective* treatment, only that the procedure would not restore the person completely.

If, for instance, a person has sustained severe brain damage, they might suggest that any treatment which would help that person live would be futile. They say this because it will never restore that person to his *original state*. Of course, when the Thanaphiles say this, they want you to believe that it means that the treatment will not work. But, what they really mean is that it will not cure *all* the problems the person has.

Modern Magicians

Judge not according to the appearance, but judge righteous judgment.

—John 7:24

Often, the complexity of the science makes the moral issues difficult to see. Looking at someone in a coma with a ventilator makes everything seem so artificial. It appears to make a difference in our decision-making capacity that this silent, unresponsive person is hooked up to machines to keep him alive. But, look past the appearance. If that ventilator was a portable unit hooked up to a person who worked two desks down from you or who lived next door and whom you often saw outside with his children, would you consider unhooking the machine? Would you call it "artificial" and "keeping him alive" in a negative way? No, you probably would marvel at the medical miracle that made it possible. If someone eventually develops a truly implantable mechanical heart, I'm sure you would feel the same way.

Why, then, does this change when someone is unresponsive to us? There is discrimination here. Based on what? It is based upon whether the person will "contribute" to society or even merely engage in social relationships. In appearance, the comatose person is different because we see no hope of return for him. This is not a Christian response—not a righteous judgment, but one based upon appearances. In God's eyes, a person's value does not depend on his abilities or contributions to society. He is made in the image of God—*imagio Dei.*

The euthanasia debate is full of technical arguments—all intended to draw our attention away from the real issues: Is the person living? How do we treat a living person? The Thanaphiles, like modern magicians, use misdirection to make it magically appear that killing people is moral and compassionate. Do not be fooled.

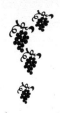

Chapter Nine

It Won't Stop with the Babies

It won't stop with the babies.
It doesn't stop with the unborn;
It doesn't stop with the babies;
Who'll be next?
Maybe you're the one![1]

As it has played out in America, abortion has been the public wedge for the entry of all sorts of death mongering. Now, it is not only the unseen unborn who are in danger, but the sickly newborn, the chronically ill, the medically dependent, the retarded, the comatose, the elderly, and an ever-growing list of people with "low quality of life."

As horrible a crime as abortion is, it does not stand alone in the list of atrocities currently practiced by the medical profession in America. There are many more as we have seen in previous chapters.

But, it is helpful to look at abortion because it shows clearly how the medical profession—and the public—bought into this wholesale slaughter of an entire class of people. It serves as a template for the other kinds of induced deaths we see occurring today.

There were several notable factors that contributed to the acceptance of abortion. First, and most important, was the abdication and silence of the Church. Second, the vacuum where the Church once stood was filled by its only competition, *paganism*. Third, language was distorted and confused so that the real issues were clouded. And finally, the mesmerizing influence of technology and arcane sciences befuddled the masses.

Before we can begin to see our way clear of this deadly morass in modern medicine, we must understand how we were subverted. Only then can we understand the road back.

Mea Culpa

> In the darkest night of our Christian church history, Hitler became for our time a marvelous transparency, a window through which light fell on the history of Christianity. . . . The aim of the Faith Movement of German Christians is an Evangelical Reich Church. Adolph [sic] Hitler's State appeals to the Church, the Church must obey the appeal.[2]

This statement was from one of the most embarrassing episodes in modern history, not just for the Christian Church, but for humanity itself. It is the statement of the German church prior to World War II—the same church that, afterwards, had to confess that it had done nothing to help the Jews or to slow, stall, or stop the mechanized killing juggernaut of Adolf Hitler.

How great a contrast from the militant Church in ages past, when Christians committed capital crimes by stealing newborns from the infanticide walls of Rome, paying for the privilege with their lives. In spite of the possibility of deadly disease, Christians cared for the sick during great plagues. At great risk, believers stood against the widow burning practice of Suttee in India, secreted away young girls who had been sold into temple prostitution, and defied English Raj law by refusing to allow tribes to continue to raise human beings like cattle to be used in human sacrifices to their blood-thirsty gods.

There are thousands of stories like this. Yet, when Germany adopted first a euthanasia program called T4 aimed at mentally deficient and physically handicapped people, little was said. When the T4 program was greatly expanded into the 14f13 program, less was said. By the time the "final solution" for racial cleansing by killing the Jews started, there was silence.

So, what happened to the German church? In many ways, her abdication of authority and courage was the result of three specific theological bases. Dietrich Bonhoeffer, a theologian and one of the founders of the Confessing Church which resisted the Third Reich, identified these perspectives.

Bonhoeffer noted the Lutheran church had adopted a world view that argued for two separate kingdoms, the world's and God's. What was valid in one realm might not be in the other, so that a Christian might operate in an arena like politics or education without any reference to the Christian ethos. And, the world itself was allowed to operate without God.

Then, there was a competing school of philosophy Bonhoeffer called Liberal Theology. Its father was Immanuel Kant, who said that Christian principles operated in a way that was detached from reality. One could pray for justice, but not try to *provide* it—except in a limited sphere like the church or the family.

The third school was called pietism. Inward perfection and devotion to God were all that was important. The world, under pietism, could just sail along to hell so long as one kept his "personal relationship with God" intact.[3]

Such heretical philosophies provided the vacuum into which nazism flowed. Can you see the comparison? The American church, beginning in the second half of the 1800s, abandoned the public arena. They simply walked away from politics, the media, the arts, medicine, and other culture-shaping positions. This, all with the misguided (not to mention Gnostic) belief that all that mattered was the soul or spirit. People were urged to enter "ministry," where ministry was solely defined by overtly "spiritually oriented" activities. Most completely excluded the ancient Christian concept of "vocation"—the idea that any work or endeavor that a Christian applied himself to was ministry. When someone distributes gospel tracts, it is called ministry. When they feed a hungry person, it is called "para-church." Such distinctions damage the full functioning of the body of Christ and denigrate some parts while vaunting others.

Today, American Christians have mostly adopted a combination of the three philosophies which were prevalent in the German church when Hitler made his political debut.

I often hear people wonder why the German church so dismally responded and, by implication, say that they would have done differently had they been there themselves. It is reminiscent of when Jesus chided the Pharisees for saying that, had they lived when their fathers did, they would not have killed the prophets as their fathers had done (Matt. 23:29–33).

I assert that the American church would have no more recognized their duty to the Jews in 1939 than they have recognized their obligation to the unborn today.

American Apathy

Many Christians today look back at the time of the founders of this nation as an era when God exerted influence in the culture and believers were free to worship in a way unparalleled in history. While some may harbor idyllic views of this time, there is much truth to that belief. America was a Christian nation.

But, what most people don't realize is that the reason God's standards had such great influence then was because God's people had been trying to exert that influence of godliness for centuries!

The German church had a wonderful history as well. They squandered their inheritance then as we squander ours today. It is our apathy that has allowed our spiritual heritage to be sucked dry. It *was* a powerful foundation, but it is not anymore.

In point of fact, such things do not exist in a vacuum. They are *purposely* brought about by the obedient, long-suffering, hard labor of the saints and the eventual response of God.

Do you long for those days? You can have them, but it will take self-sacrificing work. If your hope is that Christ will appear soon and take personal control, how will He who said, "Blessed is the servant that his lord finds so doing when he comes"[4] respond if He finds us sitting around looking at the clouds waiting for Him to do the job by Himself? Not well, I'll warrant.

After having surrendered the lead position, the American church became more and more reluctant to say anything at all about public issues. The church became irrelevant. In response to abortion, many Protestants were simply afraid of being tarred as Catholics because of the worldly perception that abortion was a "Catholic issue." The fact that Catholics were involved for years before the Protestants should cause the Protestants embarrassment. For the most part, however, Protestant and Catholic people were simply apathetic and the inertia of the proabortion movement (spawned from the pro–birth control movement)[5] resulted in massive strides in the legal and cultural acceptance of the practice.

Organized church involvement in stopping this bloodletting developed out of shame over their apathy and noninvolvement, but it was predictably "safe" and generally "too little, too late." It was reminiscent of other church efforts and the pietistic philosophy of separation—centered on the safety away from the battlefield. Just as most churches' evangelical efforts depend upon people being drawn away from their sinful influence of the world in order to hear the gospel inside a church building, so most churches involved in crisis pregnancy center work depend on women to come out of their own abortion-supporting environments and to actually seek out help to find an alternative for killing their own children. Crisis pregnancy centers are a wonderful ministry, but without a corresponding outreach into the world, they fall far short of the possibility of saving untold thousands of lives.

Few churches' activities were aimed at getting out into the world at large, either to evangelize or to protest against abortion. They mostly took the safe route. But, the CPC (Crisis Pregnancy Center) is simply not the same as going out into "the highways and hedges" in search of the lost.

The way Dr. Wolf Wolfensberger, a fighter for the lives and protection of the handicapped and a professor at the University of Syracuse, describes that the actions of the German church could easily apply to the American church.

He said their actions were:

1) slow in coming,

2) restrained in expression, and

3) just as "neat" as the extermination of the Jews in that it pursued administrative, legal and other normative channels of recourse.[6]

But, prior to the infamous *Roe vs. Wade* U.S. Supreme Court decision which legalized abortion, the American church had been so long out of a position of legal, political, and moral influence that nobody was listening when it raised its tiny peep of objection.

Vacuum

Nature, it is said, abhors a vacuum—but the devil loves one! Wherever a vacuum exists, the devil has a plan to fill it, and there has been a big void in American public life for decades (a Church-shaped void). Replacing Christianity, Satan substituted paganism. At this point, we need a working definition of paganism. As used in this work, paganism is defined in Romans 1:25. "Who changed the truth of God into a lie, and worshipped and served the creature more than the creator, who is blessed forever. Amen."

Paganism is the worship and serving of the created rather than the Creator. Whether the thing worshipped is a carved image, demon or angel, the planet, one's self, or human reason, it all amounts to paganism. The atheist is just as much the pagan as the craven idol worshipper.

By the 1950s, America had only the remnants of Christianity—an empty, civil religion. "Being religious" (at least on Sundays) had become an obligation of all "good Americans." But, it was little more than that—an obligation to polite society.

This, however, was not enough to keep the minds and hearts of men from a descent into paganism. True religion, undefiled, would have involved actual hands-on practice of Christian principles—helping the widows and fatherless—as opposed to the inactive civil religion of blind patriotism and good feelings.

The 1960s were dramatic proof that this specious religion was not sufficient to resist the forces of evil. The greatest religious explosion of the last two hundred years occurred then. Tens of thousands came to Christ in the "Jesus people" movement, and *hundreds of thousands* were converted to Eastern thought. This Eastern thought became the basis for the mass pagan thought of today's American mind. While most have not retained their connections to the New Age and Eastern cults they dabbled in back then, they retained the essential philosophies.

These young radicals of the 1960s who came to discover through their new religion that there were no absolutes and that everyone should "do their own thing," are now the doctors, lawyers, legislators, writers, artists, and journalists who shape our culture.

Small wonder that we no longer find a Christian consensus in America—much less a sympathetic hearing before official government agencies.

By the time abortion began rearing its head with new force, Christians simply lacked the credibility of an active, dynamic faith for anyone to pay attention to them. Besides, most churches were so immersed in self-centered, building-centered religion that they failed to hear the cries of the aborted calling to them for help. Others were so cowed by the prospect of facing the evil onslaught of the issue that they simply found refuge in pietism. It was not hard for Satan to replace the Church because the Church had abandoned its responsibilities and, with it, its authority was vacated.

Today, the dominant culture is no longer even marginally Christian. It is pagan—and hostile.

Euphemania

"If you call a sheep's tail a leg," Abraham Lincoln is reported to have asked a group of journalists, "How many legs would a sheep have?"

"Five," ventured one of the reporters boldly.

"No," replied Lincoln. "Four. It doesn't matter if you call a tail a leg, it's still a tail."

Words have great power. Properly used, they can elicit a response to truth. Improperly used, they can mislead and misdirect. The selection of words can enlighten or inhibit the listener. A factual statement, "He killed another man," can carry much more serious moral overtones when it is expressed, "He assassinated another man." One does not betray whether the killing was justified or not; the other expresses the idea of evil, unjustified killing. But, using other words, called euphemisms, can make what is evil appear good, such as, "He assisted another man's dignified death." Scripture tells us that God hates a false weight (Prov. 20:10, 23; Deut. 25:14). I assert that He also hates words that give ideas a false weight.

Groups of people are dehumanized (made to seem less than human) by words; the true nature of certain activities is obscured by words; and false philosophies are given credibility with false words. This is precisely what is happening in the field of medicine. And, since we are using abortion as the example, these are the very things that the pagan leaders of our culture have used to make abortion acceptable and intimidate the Church into silence about so great an evil.

Many primitive tribes call themselves by their language's equivalent of "human being." Other groups are called "dog people," "wolf people," or some other not-quite-human name. This makes killing others easier when the need or desire arises. Humans dehumanize enemies.

Black people were called "niggers." (The better to kidnap, enslave, and mistreat you with, my dear!) Jews were called "vermin." (The better to gas you, my dear!) Even legitimate enemies are easier to kill when they are given a dehumanizing name.

Americans living through World War II killed "Japs," "nips," "heines," and "krauts"—not Japanese people or German people. More recent conflicts saw "slants," "gooks," and "ragheads."

So, in abortion, we are told of "fetuses," "products of conception," and "blobs of tissue." The fact is that the child in the womb is not less human because he or she is a fetus. A fetus, like an adolescent, is simply at a stage of development. But, the proabortion culture would have us exclusively use the awkward term *fetus* in describing unborn human beings because the word tends to dehumanize them.

It should be noted that we are *all* products of conception. We were all conceived. We are merely different ages away from that conception. The terms have served their purpose well, though. Fetus, in particular, has worked because it sounds ever-so-scientific. And, Americans are intimidated by science and scientific-sounding things.

But, words are also used to obscure the real horror of evil acts. Hitler talked of a "final solution" for the Jews. In Bosnia, during the recent conflicts, we heard about "ethnic cleansing." Abortion supporters talk about "terminating a pregnancy" and "removing the products of conception." Again, words are used to obscure the truth.

Finally, words can be used to make a bad philosophy look good—or at least worthy of consideration. Look at the proabortion philosophy. The leaders of this movement scored a marketing coup when they selected the description *prochoice.*

It sounds so American, so independent, so empowering! It appeals to the selfish nature of man to believe that he (or she) should be captain of his or her own fate. But, what does the term *prochoice* really mean in the context of this debate? Is it really prochoice versus prolife?

Not really. When a child is conceived, prolife people believe in choices—keep the child or give the child up for adoption. Under the same circumstances, prochoice people believe in choices—keep the child, adopt the child out, or kill the child.

So what's the difference? Only abortion! One opposes abortion, the other favors it. Yet, the debate, conducted in a proabortion press, has maintained the idea that only prochoice people are in favor of choice.

More than that, a close examination of the activities generated by both philosophies will show that prochoice activists are rarely in favor of choices other than abortion. While prolifers open free crisis pregnancy centers (CPCs) to facilitate the choice of keeping or adopting out the child, proabortionists offer no help in such options—and often resist or deride such efforts. There are more than two thousand free CPCs in the United States, but, as far as I can determine, no free abortion clinics.

Yet, the philosophy called prochoice (because it has a positive-sounding name) is virtually immune from attack. When proabortion people say, "I'm not proabortion, I'm prochoice," most of the opposition clams up. The ploy has worked. And, the same tactic is being used to discourage us from looking too closely at many medical practices today.

The Mystique of Medicine

Science dazzles us. Medicine is a mystery. Physicians appear to be high priests—if not gods. This aura of the unknown—or unknowable—is almost religious in nature. It keeps us at arms' length in much the same way as the ancient shaman's purported magical powers kept people under control.

We are hesitant to question the decisions or advice of physicians. Medical technology has only heightened the sense of awe in which we hold medical professionals. We look at magnetic resonance imagers (MRIs) which seem to take a sideways x-ray, and shake our heads in wonder. The secrets of surgeries that apparently make problems disappear challenge our imagination.

In the abortion debate, it was not the technology or the surgical abilities which caught our attention, but the overall aura of infallibility of physicians in general. When we were told that abortions were "therapeutic"—that is, a form of medical treatment against disease—we deferred to medical judgment.

After *Roe vs. Wade*, we generally thought that there would be few abortions and that they were going to be performed only when dire circumstances warranted it.

Nor were many other medical "advances" questioned because of our fascination with the amazing feats of science involved. We were so busy being captivated by what medicine was *able* to do, that we never bothered to ask *whether* certain things *should* be done.

Doctors, also, appear to be above us. Their knowledge and experience seems to place them in another realm where their judgment on medical matters is beyond question.

Of course, this is not true. You have the same ability—and obligation—to look into the facts before making medical decisions as you have before making serious financial decisions. You should ask questions, questions, questions, until you understand and are satisfied, then you should get a second and third opinion.

It Didn't Stop with the Babies

There are three things that are never satisfied, yea, four that say not, It is enough. The grave . . .
—Proverbs 30:15–16

Truly, death does not say, "It is enough" in America—not even in the case of medically caused (or iatrogenic) death.

As we see elsewhere in this book, the philosophy of death has taken over the medical world in the West and produces more and more varieties of abomination. There is a spiritual component as well, which will also be discussed in a later chapter. The spirit of the one who comes to steal, kill, and destroy is behind it—even when the participants do not even believe in a spiritual realm. But, a surprising number of the leading Thanaphiles do see their activities as a spiritual quest and openly acknowledge it in shockingly candid statements.

You see, the battle between Darkness and Light does not confine itself to the soul and the spirit. The body is an integral part of our created being.

All that it touches—work, family, community, politics—is part of the battlefield as well. It is a war between two world views. There is no pluralism possible. Only one side can win.

Medicine is no different. Either it will be guided by Christian principles or it will be guided by pagan principles. The two meet every day in the hospitals and clinics of this country. We, as Christians, must begin to impose a Christ-centered world view on these institutions—even if only where we are responsible for the medical decisions of ourselves or others. Our decisions must be informed by a Christian world view.

First, however, we must explore the two world views—Christian and pagan. What presumptions do each of these ideologies operate under? What difference does it make? That, we shall look at in the next chapter.

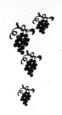

Chapter Ten

Christian vs. Pagan Ethics: Battle of the Radicals

If you are a Christian, your ideas are radical. The same is true of the pagan. We all live according to radical ideas. Radical, meaning "from the center" or "from the heart," is the essence of all core beliefs. And, ideas have consequences. Whatever you truly believe, you will act upon.

The reason you feel the wall inside a doorway when you enter a dark room is that you truly believe that by simply finding and flicking a switch, the room will be flooded with light. You act on this belief almost without thinking. The reason you pray when no one else can see or hear you is because you believe there is a God who hears you.

"Ideas have consequences" is only a reiteration of the Master's teachings, "If you love Me, you will keep my commandments" and "You will know them by their fruits."[1] If someone does not keep His commandments, he does not love Christ, notwithstanding his loudest protestations. If the "fruits" of a man's life indicate that he believes in the me-first philosophy, you will know what his core beliefs are.

Both Christians and pagans act out of core beliefs, and there is a battle between the two. The field of medicine is one of the major battlegrounds.

In order to discern from which set of core beliefs the "new" medical ethics flow, we must examine—side by side—some of the presumptions and core beliefs of both. Before we do, however, an explanation of medical ethics is in order.

The Medical Ethics Garden

These bioethicists . . . have gardens in which they cultivate only euphemisms.
                  —Nat Hentoff, editor of *Village Voice*

Medical ethics, in the way the term is currently used, bears the impression that *medical* ethics are somehow different from other *ethics*. The use of the word *ethics* also implies that there was a moral decision-making process and that the conclusions are sound. This impression is not true. Originally, medical ethics was simply how common Christian morality, or ethics, was applied to the singular practices and issues faced in medicine.

But, because of the purported complexity of modern medicine, it is proposed that medical ethics can be different from the ethics we nonmedical people are expected to live by. It is small wonder that some physicians develop god complexes. They think they are above ordinary rules governing mankind.

I believe that God foresaw modern medicine's predicaments and supplied us with all we need to make rational, moral decisions. And, moral decisions—Christian morality—are ultimately *rational*.

As much as the pagans would like to convince you that only *their* core ideas are scientific and reasonable, this is not the case.

Christian ideas are so rational that even secular governments use them as the bases of law. Even some atheists, like Nat Hentoff quoted above, are convinced to become prolife because of the ultimate rationality of the Christian precept of respect for *all* human life.

As we compare the competing ideas of Christianity with the pagan ideas, remember that not all pagans think alike. Some, for instance, believe their lives are foreordained by the stars or fate, while others believe in absolute free will (as noted later). However, these seemingly opposite beliefs are both pagan and do not acknowledge God—they are creation-centered, not Creator-centered.

But, a close look at the competing beliefs will enable us to see the motivations behind many of the so-called medical ethics of today and how the medical profession is able to justify some of the worst abominations ever devised by man.

Some of the competing core beliefs might be listed as follows:

Christian	Pagan
1. God is sovereign.	Man (or nature) is sovereign.
2. You shall not shed innocent blood.	Man, innocent or not, is expendable.
3. All men are created equal.	Some men are more valuable than others.

4. Care for the infirm, the elderly, and the needy.	Survival of the fittest.
5. Man is created in God's image.	Man is an animal.
6. Right and wrong are absolutes.	Situation ethics/there are no absolutes.
7. God's Word is the only Truth.	All beliefs are equal.
8. Obey God.	Do your own thing.
9. Love one another.	The betterment of society.
10. It is given once to die, then judgment.	Annihilation, higher planes, or reincarnation.

Who Is Sovereign?

"My body, my choice," screams the pro-abortion crowd, the pro-suicide crowd, and the pro-homosexuality crowd.

Just about everyone is screaming these days. Everyone wants to do whatever they want so long as it does not "harm others." The man suffering some incurable disease wants to commit suicide and wants the help of his doctor and others to do it. "Whose life is it anyway?" he asks. The argument makes a lot of sense to the average person. After all, they think, as long as he isn't hurting anyone else . . .

But, the belief that God is sovereign is a core belief of Christians, and the belief that man is sovereign is a pagan belief. Admittedly, some pagans believe in fate or destiny, or that the gods control their every move, but none of those approach the idea of the sovereignty of God. In Christianity, man has free will, but God is sovereign. In this case, He has said that the time of life and death is one area where He is absolute.

However, evidence that most of the world's population chooses to believe that man is sovereign appears most clearly in the discussions over medical technology. "We can keep a person's body alive almost indefinitely," they say trying to ratchet up the horror of the audience over being "kept alive by machines." But, they flatter themselves.

The Scriptures plainly say that God is the Lord over life and death, that He has numbered our days. How arrogant of anyone to think that they, a mere human, could possibly keep anyone alive longer than God would allow.

We have discussed the actual, as opposed to the fanciful, abilities of medical technology in keeping people alive. Suffice it to say that all of our medical technology can only assist the body to function temporarily. A ventilator, for instance, can pump air into lungs, but if the lungs no longer oxygenate blood, it is fruitless. Yes, without the assistance, a *living* person might die, but if the vital organs stop doing all of what they are supposed to do, no machine will keep that body going.

Scripture tells us that none of us lives or dies unto ourselves. Whether or not we want to admit it, we all have an obligation to fulfill the will of God—Christian and pagan alike. We also have duties to our family, friends, neighbors, and communities that should prevent us from doing what we like with our own bodies.

Innocent Blood

Perhaps no single precept better encapsulates the basis for how Christians are to treat other people than the concept of innocent blood. It is the basis for laws against murder, human sacrifice, cannibalism, and even the system of justice that presumes innocence and prohibits punishment of people until guilt is proven. It also prohibits killing people "for the good of society," "for their own good," because they are "too expensive," or because "they do not live up to our expectations." The shedding of innocent blood is categorically prohibited in Scripture.

Pagan thought, on the other hand, permits the killing of innocent people for various reasons. Ancient human sacrifices were done for the good of society. The Chinese Book of Rites says that human sacrifice "has as its main aim to bring back social union and to restore the cosmic order."[2] Such sentiments are not uncommon. Many societies sacrificed their firstborn children in order to procure future fertility. Others did so for better crops or in hopes of future prosperity.

Similarly, so are abortion and euthanasia performed in today's society. The only difference is the religious trappings. The ancient priest wore feathers and beads and the modern priest wears surgical garb.

Equality Versus Graded Value

We are all equal, except that some are more equal than others.

—George Orwell

It took centuries for the biblical concept of human equality to come through in both philosophical and governmental arenas. The American experiment was one of the first major manifestations of what Scripture had said all along—that all men were equal in the sight of God and should be equal in the sight of the law. Even the Law of Moses prohibited having "one law for the Israelite and another for the stranger" (Exod. 12:49; Num. 15:16).

Since ancient times, however, nobility have always been regarded as above the mass of humanity. Pagan ideals held most rulers to have some of the divine in them. An offense against one of them was a much greater crime than the same offense against a common man. An offense by them, particularly against someone of lower status, was regarded as a mere trifle—or, in some cases, no offense at all.

In today's pagan mind, the measure consists of whether the person can be expected to contribute to society financially or in some other measurable way, or if they have any social relationships that bind them to the community and the community to them. Of course, the unborn, particularly if judged to be in danger of a low quality of life, do not qualify as equal to the mother who has social relationships and a voice to assert her "rights." The comatose or brain dead need not apply. The right of the retarded to live is certainly in question.

Good Samaritans and Survivalists

If the physician presumes to take into consideration in his work whether a life has value or not, the conse-

quences are boundless and the physician becomes the most
dangerous man in the state.
        —Dr. Christoph Hufeland (1762–1836)

If there is anything that has become the ear-
mark of modern medicine, it is the idea that a doctor should determine the value of the life of his
patient before considering treatment. In this way,
doctors can ration treatment to those who would
truly benefit from it and essentially cull the weak
from the human herd.

Over a century ago, Charles Darwin popular-
ized a pagan notion that the survival of the fittest
was the selection process by which humanity and all
other forms of life advance. It was not a new idea.
The concept of the "divine right of kings" and the
practices of "trial by combat" and "trial by ordeal"
all had their basis in that premise. Might makes
right!

Today's hospitals are full of talk about such ideas.
I recall the time after I had my first heart attack. I
was seated with my doctor, who was urging me to
submit to a coronary bypass operation. I was resisting the suggestion. "Mr. deParrie," he said, in his
best imitation of a voice of concern, "we would not
have even offered this treatment if you weren't so
young and in otherwise good health."

Without the faintest idea of what he had said to
me, the doctor had spoken volumes about his core
beliefs and what he perceived his job to be. Not
only had he clearly based his offer of treatment on
his personal evaluation of whether or not I would
contribute to society, but he had determined that
my value was just high enough to make me worthy

of survival. Clearly, he was saying that he would have never even *offered* a life-saving treatment to me if I had not measured up to his standard of fitness or worthiness.

This doctor was not my physician, such as I had had when I was a child, one that would come out in the middle of the night to serve his patient. This doctor was a social engineer, determining just how many and what kind of people should be allowed to survive—which people would help society to survive. While in Darwin's scheme of things, the predators culled out the weakest of the prey, allowing the strongest to survive; with humans, we act as our own predators.

Where the Scripture commands us to care for the sick, as it does in Matthew 10:8 (not to kill them), and two thousand years of Christian medical ethics have called physicians to be a sacrificial profession (ministry) focused on the needs of the patient before them, pagan ethics now call upon doctors to dispassionately evaluate the worthiness of patients to receive care and the possible financial and social impact of their continued existence.

Special

"I am not an animal!"

This cry was one of the most profound and moving moments of both the play and the movie, *Elephant Man*. While the press and the public generally touted the story and highlighted that very quote, the message has apparently not sunk in.

Consider the euthanasia debate. One of the most common arguments for euthanasia is that we "put down" our pets and other animals when they are very sick, so why not people? This lowers the value of a human to that of an animal. The words of Peter Singer, noted medical philosopher and writer, are chilling:

> Once the religious mumbo-jumbo surrounding the term "human" has been stripped away, we may continue to see normal members of our species as possessing greater capacities of rationality, self-consciousness, communication, and so on, than members of other species; but we will not regard as sacrosanct the life of each and every member of our species, no matter how limited its capacity for intelligent or even conscious life may be. . . . Only the fact that the defective infant is a member of the species Homo Sapiens leads it to be treated differently from a dog or pig. Species membership alone, however, is not morally relevant. Humans who bestow superior value on the lives of all human beings solely because they are members of our own species, are judging along lines strikingly similar to those used by white racists.[3]

And, this was what he was saying in 1983! Certainly, the animal rights crowd—those who protest for "rights" to be given to animals—approach this from the opposite direction. They elevate animals to the level of humans. Rodney A. Coronado, an animal rights activist, recently pled guilty to bombing an animal research facility in Michigan after freeing its inhabitants.[4] The media was full of sympathetic coverage for a man "committed to his cause."

In whatever way we may treat an animal, we may treat a human. Also, there is no special significance to human beings.

God says differently. He created man in His own image and endowed him with the ability to have a relationship with God and to dwell with God forever. For this reason alone, man must be treated differently. No animal has such abilities or promise. Nor does any animal have the responsibilities of a man. Man, not animals, will face judgment for the deeds done during his life.

Since man's physical body is an integral part of creation—and made in the image of God—it matters how we treat it. Orthodox Jews will not even allow autopsies on their dead because it will defile that image. Early Christians were arrested and even executed when they retrieved the bodies of slaves thrown away in the Roman dumps in order to give them a proper burial. Why would they take such risks? Because those slaves were made in God's image and even their dead bodies deserved greater respect than being tossed in the dump. Man is not an animal, and under no circumstances should he be treated as one.

Absolutely No Absolutes

Without a holy (separate from creation) God or a judgment to come, there can be no absolutes. It would be utterly foolish to believe in them or act on any kind of morality if one were, say, an atheist or a believer in reincarnation. Eat, drink, and be merry, for tomorrow we die! Do whatever you can get away with!

Most pagans, however, are reluctant to follow the ultimate logic of their beliefs. They settle for a cross between situation ethics, right and wrong being determined by the circumstances, and sentimental, emotion-borne ideas about what is "appropriate" (their favorite word used to avoid calling things right or wrong) and what is not.

They will maintain that there are no absolutes, but, when questioned closely, they will list many absolutes. Ask them about racism or molesting two-year-olds. Then ask them on what they base this morality which they would wish to "impose" on everyone.

Bertrand Russell, an avowed atheist and early 20th century philosopher, saw through the situation ethics argument. "If good and bad," he said, "are determined by whether the results are good or bad, how do we know whether the results are good or bad?" In other words, if there are no absolutes, then we have no gauge to measure the results.

Stranger yet, the same people who assert there are no absolutes have very definite ideas about what is right and wrong—ideas that often are ironically based in Christian morality. They believe in human equality (except when it gets inconvenient), being truthful (except when it gets in the way of what they want), caring for the less fortunate (except when it gets in the way), and dozens of other Christian-based ideals.

However, God has some very stodgy ideas of His own. He says, as we have already mentioned, that we may never "shed innocent blood" (Deut. 19:10). He tells us we may never commit fornication or adultery. Certainly, there are times when God's Word shows us that we may do some things under extreme circumstances that we are otherwise not to do. The lies told by the Hebrew midwives, Esther, and Rahab the harlot were examples. Disobedience to civil authority seen in the Book of Acts and throughout the Scriptures constitutes another area. But, the "rules," as it were, for these kinds of deviations are discoverable in Scripture. God, however, made no exceptions to some laws. Those laws, too, are discoverable in His Word.

The Pluralism Game

> *Let God be true, but every man a liar.*
> —Romans 3:4

Pluralism is the belief that all religions or belief systems not only have the same right to be heard but are equal in stature. While the concept of pluralism has gained wide acceptance, its premise is fairly easily refuted. I am aware of no one who would agree that the belief that the earth is flat is as worthy of acceptance as the belief in a spherical earth. Some belief systems manifestly produce misery and poverty. Christianity teaches compassion for the less fortunate and has produced hospitals and outreaches to feed and clothe people.

Only God's Word claims ultimate Truth. Other religions usually claim that there are many paths to God, but that theirs is the best. However, the true spirit of paganism is revealed once it gains ascendancy. Suddenly, pluralism is only a virtue if you are in agreement with the pagans. Christianity always becomes the target because it is "intolerant"—

it claims the only true way is Jesus Christ. This is precisely what got the early Christians in the worst trouble with Rome. Rome had controlled most of the known world by promoting the idea of diversity and accepted the concept of syncretism in religion—that is, that "all religions basically teach the same thing." (Where have we heard *that* before?)

But, a religion that claimed to be the only way was not to be tolerated. In medicine today, we are told to accept decisions that others make which result in the death of the unborn or the comatose. We are told that the person deciding is following their own religious beliefs. In fact, "their own religious beliefs" often refers to the mindset of the pagan social engineers. Yet, as we shall see, when Christians attempt to exercise their own religious beliefs in making medical decisions to save those lives, the hospitals fight tooth and nail.

Obey God or Obey Self

Different strokes for different folks.
Do your own thing.
Follow your heart.
Harming no other, do what you will.
Do whatever works for you.
I have the right to do whatever I want as long as
*   I don't hurt anyone else.*
No one else can tell you what is right for you.

These are all expressions of the same thing—a belief that each man is sufficient unto himself to decide what is right and wrong. It is the basis of the "values clarification" teaching which infests the public schools. It was the groundwork of the hippie movement of the 1960s. It is the general philosophy of Wicca (Western European witchcraft) and the foundation of "non-judgmental, total-acceptance, non-directive" psychology. And, it is the running theme of all of those touchy-feely afternoon talk shows on television.

There is the pretense that "doing your own thing" is somehow mitigated by the "doing no harm" or "as long as I don't hurt anyone else" part of the equation, but it never really works.

Why? Because not only are you deciding what is good for you, but you also get to decide what constitutes harm to others. Since no one agrees on these basic questions, the real philosophy boils down to do whatever you want that you can get away with. Does anyone want to be on the rules committee of *that* anarchists' convention? God, however, demands obedience to Him—and that you do *His* thing.

People or Society

Jesus, ever practical, gave us very simple marching orders—orders that dealt with immediate problems. He told us to love our neighbor, not to love everyone in the whole world. He told us to feed the hungry, not to found an organization that we hoped would feed the world's hungry by the year 2001.

Loving (or feeding) the whole world, as admirable as that might be, is not possible for us as human beings. Jesus wants us to love the people we meet. Actually, it is much easier to "love" the whole world than it is to love that irritating guy you work with or that woman who lives next door. It is simpler to have loving feelings about an amorphous mass of humanity than to deal with the peculiarities of people we know. So, Jesus has commanded us to do the real thing and love our neighbor.

Pagans, on the other hand, are always going on about "the betterment of society." With this object in mind, they can casually ration health care to people "who truly need it" in the name of the greatest good for the greatest number. Their focus is on "loving" that amorphous mass of humanity at the expense of trampling a sick or dying person right in front of them. They are, like my doctor mentioned earlier, social engineers.

The old medical ethic was concerned about the "neighbor" (patient) at hand. It was based upon the command to love one another. The new medical ethic is willing to "love" society by withholding medical care from you in order to have it available to someone more worthy—someone who will best benefit society.

The Last Enemy

Man was never meant to die. God made him to be immortal. But, since the Fall, there has been death and death is the very door to our judgment and final reward. Though, for believers, our physical deaths lead to our reward, the Scripture's view of death is that it is an enemy.

"The last enemy that shall be destroyed is death," says 1 Corinthians 15:26.

This enemy is overcome in the resurrection, when we, once again, have a body. At this time, we will become what we were originally intended to be—immortal—and more! While physical life should not become a god, the Scriptures do not leave a lot of room for befriending death.

But, the pagan medical view of death is that it is "part of life," natural, and, therefore, good. To pagans, it represents a simple ending or annihilation of the person, or, for the religiously inclined, a doorway into reincarnation or a higher, better plane. In this view, there is no reason to avoid death.

Scripture tells us that it is given to man once to die, and then the judgment (Heb. 9:27). But, the pagan view sees no judgment—at least no hell or punishment. This leaves pagans with little reason to avoid using death as a solution to problems. The physician-assisted suicide movement reflects this philosophy.

Three Steps

Having looked briefly at the major philosophical differences between Christian and pagan thought related to medical ethics, we still need to understand the medical issues. There are generally three steps to making moral decisions:

1) Knowing what the Word of God says
2) Knowing what the facts are
3) Prayer

Often, prayer is not specifically needed when the commands of Scripture are clear. No one needs to pray about whether to murder someone. For instance, once someone understands that abortion is the shedding of innocent blood, there is no need to pray about whether or not to have an abortion. But, in the field of medicine, there is a lot of mys-

tery, a lot of smoke and mirrors, and a lot of deliberate deception.

Deliberate deception? Yes, as early as 1970, three
years before the legalization of abortion by the U.S.
Supreme Court, the prestigious journal, *California
Medicine: The Western Journal of Medicine*, wrote
quite boldly about its use of misdirected language
and euphemisms in order to soften opposition to
doctors killing people.

> The traditional Western ethic has always
> placed great emphasis on the intrinsic worth
> and equal value of every human life regard-
> less of its stage or condition. . . .
>
> There are certain new facts and social reali-
> ties which are becoming widely recognized,
> and are widely discussed in Western society
> and seem certain to undermine and trans-
> form this traditional ethic. . . .
>
> Since the old [Judeo-Christian] ethic has not
> yet been fully displaced it has been necessary
> to separate the idea of abortion from the
> idea of killing, which continues to be so-
> cially abhorrent. The result has been a curi-
> ous avoidance of the scientific fact, which
> everyone really knows, that human life be-
> gins at conception and is continuous whether
> intra- or extra-uterine until death. The very
> considerable semantic gymnastics which are
> required to rationalize abortion as anything
> but taking a human life would be ludicrous
> if they were not often put forth under so-
> cially impeccable auspices.[5]

This article concludes that similar "semantic
gymnastics" put forth by doctors (under socially im-

peccable auspices) will be needed when we have moved on from "birth control and birth selection" to the more daunting task of "death control and death selection."

But, more important, consider the arrogant attitude of this writer. Clearly, he believes that man is no more than an animal—and *less*, if he doesn't measure up to Peter Singer's standards. It is not surprising to note that Singer, quoted earlier in the chapter, looms very large in current times in the animal rights movement.

Why Are They Here?

Like so many things that we face, our big question seems to be, "Why?" In this case, I am talking about the retarded, the comatose, and the other dependent people we have in our midst. Why are they here?

I suggest they are here to test *our* humanity. The Scriptures often tell us to comfort the afflicted, defend the fatherless, assist the poor, visit the widow—in other words, to supply whatever help we can to people who are dependent through no fault of their own. We are certainly not told to assist the lazy or foolish. But, why not tell us to defend the rights of the middle class and to visit the wealthy? After all, they are the ones "who make America work." They are the salt-of-the-earth types. It is not that God is not interested in these people—He is, but He wants us to practice seeing His image in others. He wants us to see His image in "the least of these." He wants us to see this for two reasons. First, because it is a fact that they are made in His image, and, second, because it is *difficult* to see them that way.

Human nature dictates that we only acknowledge those who can help us, but God says otherwise. The poor and afflicted are in the same straits as the medically dependent—they cannot help themselves, and they need the help of others. We will never know whether we will obey the commands of Christ to feed the hungry, clothe the naked, comfort the afflicted, and defend the fatherless and widow until we face our neighbors in need and extend ourselves to help them.

Like the Good Samaritan, we are to help those in need. It not only helps those in need, it makes *us* conform more to His image when we help those who are also in His image. It is a matter of your core beliefs—a matter of living for the One you believe is your Lord.

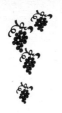

Chapter Eleven

Moral Murder

As society progresses in a spiral, we will again come to see the higher morality of destroying the unfit.[1]
—Karl Binding, professor
of law and philosophy

Evidently, society has "progressed in a spiral" quite a bit since this quote first appeared in *Permitting the Destruction of Unworthy Life* in Germany in the 1920s. Today, compassion, morality, and religious reasons are often asserted for killing. It has always been so.

Human sacrifice, as discussed in an earlier chapter, has almost always been rooted in one or another form of religious expression. Remember the words of Nigel Davies when discussing the basis for the practice? "The underlying conditions did not alter: lack of any benevolent redeemer, absence of a truly humane ethic, and, finally, belief in a ceaseless cycle of rebirth that turned the death of man into a trivial incident." But, there were, he says, commingled, practical effects: "The custom of human sacrifice admits that the life of one is taken to save the lives of many, or that of an inferior individual is put to death for the purpose of preventing the death of somebody who has a higher right to live."[2]

"Higher morality," "benevolent redeemer," "higher right to live"—these are *religious* concepts. But, religion does not always appear religious. Many of the ancients worshiped their gods not as actual beings but representative ideals to be sought after. Often we will see essentially the same concepts a religion holds played out in a more secular-looking way. A good example is the theory of evolution. This is nothing more than the scientific version of creation as told by myriads of ancient pagan cultures.[3] In old times, infants were sometimes sacrificed to gods and goddesses to ensure future prosperity. Today, abortions are obtained by mothers for the sake of their own future prosperity. There is little difference—especially from the perspective of the sacrificial victim.

Had an Aztec simply reached out to a neighbor and cut him open and taken his heart, I'm certain he would have been accused of murder. But, make the man a priest (a sacred profession) and put him on top of the temple mound (a sacred place), and suddenly the same act is transformed into not only a legal act, but one that is actually praised.

Now, have a person decide to stop feeding his grandmother who lives in his home, and the media would have no end of hand-wringing over what a beast the man was. Make the man a doctor (the sacred profession) with the woman in a hospital (the sacred place), and he will be described as courageous and compassionate. Those who would try to stop this death by starvation would be called busybodies and moralists trying to cram their morality down other people's throats and "play God."

Like the Nazi doctors in the German euthanasia program, the Thanaphiles have thoroughly medicalized the killing so that it is beyond reproach. The virtual supernaturalization of all that is scientific shields the decisions of today's medical ethicists from serious inquiry.

Scientism and the Great American Medical Priesthood

Doctors are really the priests of the Church of Modern Medicine.[4]

—The late Dr. Robert Mendelsohn, former chairman of the Medical Licensing Committee for the State of Illinois and a critic of the medical profession

It is no surprise to anyone that Americans worship in a scientific church. The ultimate answers to life, Americans believe, can be found in science— Where do we come from? Why are we here? Where are we going? Is there anything outside of this universe? All these and more, the priest of scientism seeks to answer.

But, most Americans have little or no access to the higher level of priests—the ones who study quantum physics and such. However, they are usually content with their contacts with psychologists, psychiatrists, and medical doctors. These appear to be able to help us to apply ultimate truths to our daily lives. These can show us the way to be healthy and happy.

Even those who deviate from the standards—those who use meditation, reflexology, and dozens of other alternatives—do so based upon allegedly scientific proof that their method works. In fact, the practitioners of most New Age or occultic religions in the United States spend a great deal of time trying to prove the rational and scientific basis for their activities. They go so far as to make the supernatural realm into just another plane of the natural realm. This appeals to the American mind.

With this in mind, it is easy to see how Americans now view doctors and psychologists with the same type of mystical awe that used to be reserved for priests and shamans in older, more primitive cultures. It might also be noted that, in most primitive cultures, the role of priests included medicine. It matters little whether medicine takes on religious trappings, so long as it fills the sacred place that religion fills. As I have noted above, ordinarily horrendous acts can be justified if they are done by the "sacred person" in the "sacred place" and for "sanctified reasons." As the Scriptures say, there is nothing new under the sun. As the current vernacular goes, the more things change, the more they stay the same.

Things under the Sun

As I pursued the work, it became clear that the Nazis were not the only ones to involve doctors in evil. One only need look at the role of Soviet psychiatrists in diagnosing dissenters as mentally ill and incarcerating them in mental hospitals: of doctors in Chile (as documented by Amnesty International) serving as torturers;

of Japanese doctors performing medical experiments and vivisection on prisoners during the second World War; of South African doctors falsifying medical reports of blacks tortured or killed in prison; of American physicians and psychologists employed by the Central Intelligence Agency in the recent past for unethical medical and psychological experiments involving drugs and mind manipulation; and of the "idealistic" young physician-member of the People's Temple cult in Guyana preparing the poison (a mixture of cyanide and Kool-Aid) for the combined murder-suicide in 1978 of almost a thousand people.[5]

—Robert Jay Lifton, M.D.

The quote above only includes this century's abuse of the medical practice, but remember that once, in ancient times, *all* physicians were healer/poisoners. And, even since the advent of the Christianized Hippocratic system, there have always been those who corrupted the medical arts for their own gain. Science and medicine are too powerful a tool for fallen man not to pervert.

So, the Nazis were not alone, but the Nazi doctors are an easy target. They left records of their deeds. That is why they are used so often. But, the fact is that humanity has always been just as corruptible as it was in Germany. It is simply easier to document the German medical holocaust.

At first, after World War II, people were numbed by the sheer magnitude of what the Nazis had done. Later, however, it became apparent that the Nazis were more than crazed, bloodthirsty monsters. They were systematic, organized, deliberate procurers of what one man called a "bureaucratic, spic-and-span hell." All the careful recording of each of the bureaucratic murders—millions of them—made studying the depths of this depravity much easier for ethicists and historians. It was in this study where the most shocking discovery of the Holocaust was made—that without the cooperation of the medical community, the Nazis could never have pulled it off. "Auschwitz was like a medical operation," one Holocaust survivor said. "The killing program was led by doctors from beginning to end."[6]

Germans back then were like Americans today in their worship of science. The authoritarian German culture allowed for the mass shipping of people to death camps in a way that would not yet be possible in America, but it was the air of medical authority (the sacred person) that lent legitimacy to the killings themselves.

And, like all religions, medicine has its own sacred emblems. Chief among them is the priestly "vestment" of the white lab coat. The Nazis did not overlook the power of this image in people's minds. When they transported the "unfit" mental patients and handicapped people to the centers where they were to be euthanized, they took advantage of this powerful, justifying totem.

> SS personnel manned the buses, frequently wearing white uniforms or white coats in order to appear to be doctors, nurses, or medical attendants. There were reports of "men with white coats and SS boots," the combination that epitomized much of the "euthanasia" project in general.[7]

Nor have such symbols lost their power in modern times. Dr. Pieter Admiraal, a noted Dutch Thanaphile, is known to remove his white coat when giving a patient a lethal injection. In a medical ethics symposium in 1994, Dr. John M. Dolan pointed out that this was probably a reflex response to Admiraal's training as a physician, showing his internal discomfort with the idea that a doctor would kill. Others, however, continue to use what could only be called useless medical religious rituals in times like this. One doctor is described this way when killing a patient. "Alone in a bedroom with his patient, [Dr.] Burghard carefully swabbed the injection site, falling back on basic medical training that teaches respect for the human body so complete that even an injection intended to kill must be preceded by the normal preparations."[8]

Strangely, we see the same thing in an Auschwitz survivor's description of the infamous Nazi doctor, Josef Mengele, as he gave deadly phenol injections to kill prisoners. "Mengele then rubbed alcohol on the spot, just under the elbow, that he was using for the injection, and then injected the phenol. . . . He did it as though he were performing regular surgery."[9]

Modern Medicine's Doctrines

The lead quote for this chapter stated that destroying the unfit was a "higher morality." Much of this kind of doctrine is based upon evolution. Strangely enough, many Eastern mystic and what we call New Age religions hold similar tenets. Maharishi Mahesh Yogi has said,

There has not been and there will not be a
place for the unfit. The fit will lead, and if
the unfit are not coming along, there is no
place for them. . . . In the Age of enlightenment there is no place for ignorant people.
Nature will not allow ignorance to prevail. It
just can't. Non-existence of the unfit has been
the law of nature.[10]

This is actually a restatement of the Darwinian
principle of survival of the fittest. The Marharishi's
comments were directed at the *spiritually* unfit not
being allowed to exist in the "age of enlightenment."
But, this is not very encouraging. The question
might be asked: Who decides which people are
spiritually fit and what do we do about those who
are not?

The Nazis, as mystical and occultic as their doctrines were, based their decisions of fitness on physical attributes and abilities or race. They also believed that "non-existence of the unfit has been the
law of nature." We all know how they disposed of
those regarded as unfit.

Such similarities are not accidental. I believe
that they all flow from the same spirit. Each may
have a different outworking, but the doctrine is the
same. Whether expressed by the Darwinian, the
Nazi, or the New Ager, it is all the same teaching—
the strong survive.

Currently we see this mentality reflected in organizations like Planned Parenthood, March of
Dimes, and the Rockefeller Foundation. The study
of eugenics, the attempt to improve the gene pool
of human beings, has slowly returned. More and
more, we hear leading public figures and medical

ethicists talk of eliminating hereditary diseases—by eliminating the diseased.

Often infused into the evolutionary survival of the fittest mentality is the view of society as a single organism where the individual becomes unimportant. The Germans called it *Volk*—the folks, the people, the race—and geared their whole medical society toward the health of the *Volk*. That was the rationale behind the euthanasia program against the physically and mentally "unfit" and, later, the elimination of the Jews and other "infections" of the Nordic race.

In fact, the German doctors came to believe what Karl Binding, quoted at the beginning of the chapter, said—that the weakening of the Nordic race was due to Christianity-inspired "erroneous thinking" about "ballast-type people." Binding wrote:

> A long and painful development [of the higher morality of killing the unfit] over the centuries has been retarded partly because of the Christian way of thinking which has brought us to our present way of thinking.
>
> A new time will come when we no longer in the name of higher morality will carry out this demand that has its origin in an exaggerated idea of humanity.
>
> The present morality places too much value on mere continuation of existence and asks too high a sacrifice.[11]

"Exaggerated idea of humanity?" This sounds very much like our earlier quote of a modern medical ethicist, Peter Singer, who spoke about the "religious mumbo-jumbo" surrounding human life.

Binding's quote may have been made in the 1920s, but he has many powerful doctrinal descendants. People are no longer individuals valuable in and of themselves. They become cells in an organism to be used when needed and cast off when they have lost their value. Recall our quote from Dr. Richard Baily: "Human life has economic value only as a function of its ability to produce goods and services that are demanded by others."

Note how often today we hear talk of people as human resources and about the lack of medical resources for society. One doctor testified in court regarding Baby Ryan, mentioned in an earlier chapter, that Ryan, if he continued to live, would "contaminate society." Such statements are understandable based upon the doctrines of survival of the fittest and the search to improve humanity as a whole. When a doctor is more concerned about the overall health of society or about whether medical resources are sufficient for the entire society, he has fallen into the trap of treating mankind and not the individual before him as the patient. He has become a social engineer for the American version of the Volk. From there, it is only a baby step to justifying the killing of "unfit" patients for the good of society.

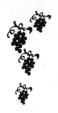

Chapter Twelve

The Very Ideas

Ideas have consequences.

—Richard Weaver

Thought precedes action. And, the kinds of thoughts we think—even subconsciously—will influence what *kinds* of actions we take. So it is with our medical decisions, particularly those medical decisions we make on behalf of others. Our thinking about these medically dependent people will eventually shape the treatment they receive, whether unto life or unto death. And, this thinking comes under many influences. The subtle voices of "reason" of the medical staff, the drubbing, continuous murmur of the ideas implanted through the media, and the internal confusion created by euphemisms and distorted words all come to bear on our minds when these difficult decisions become ours.

Emotions also play a major role in manipulating euthanasia. The high tension and feelings of love for the patient can often be distorted to make killing appear compassionate or even beneficial. This is why it is important to understand the situation accurately, to know the applicable biblical precepts, and to clearly articulate well-founded beliefs before the situation arises.

Compassion Fascists

"I wouldn't want to live like that."

We've all said it before. We've all looked at someone with a disability, or an illness, or a condition that impairs their daily lives and we've said it. It is perfectly natural for those of us in reasonably good health not to want to lose it. We find it hard to imagine living with limited abilities—physical or mental—or in pain or dependent on others for simple needs. Nobody *wants* to live that way—even those who do. But, this is an entirely different question than whether we would *adjust* to living that way or whether we would (when the chips were down) rather *die* than live that way.

The Thanaphiles know we all feel this way, and they play on that. This mechanism is one of the most common for promoting their ends. The argument is a distortion of the do-unto-others-as-you-would-have-them-do-unto-you command of Scripture. First, you are made to see or visualize the pitiful picture of a person severely handicapped, gravely ill, or in excruciating pain. The I'd-hate-to-have-to-live-like-*that* reflex kicks in immediately. From there, it is not hard for them to tug on your empathy and compassion for the person and slip in the question of whether they might not be "better off dead" than enduring this suffering.

The supporters of euthanasia talk understandingly of the suffering the person is undergoing and how life has become a burden—though to listen carefully to them, one might think the patient himself is the burden. Our overreaction to the idea of suddenly going from having full use of our faculties to being in the condition of our poor subject makes it almost certain that we can safely answer yes.

Voila! Killing becomes an act of compassion. The Second Great Commandment of Christ, you shall love your neighbor as yourself, gets turned on end. The Second Great Commandment is actually turned *against* the First Commandment (to love God with your whole heart, soul, and mind), in that you must sin against God by shedding innocent blood in order to "obey" the Second Commandment in an exercise of false compassion.

Oddly, our protestations aside, most people do adjust to and accept these conditions of disability and heightened dependence on others when they are thrust upon them. The suicide rate among retarded individuals, for instance, is very low. We feel sorrier for them than they feel for themselves. College students—especially medical students—have extremely high suicide rates. But, even those who express a desire for suicide among the infirm, elderly, and severely handicapped are known to be depressed. They often feel abandoned by friends and family. Or, they are made to feel like they and their medical expenses are a burden. When those issues are resolved, they rarely ask for death.

Often, the death of a person is presented as "for their own good." This old saw has been used for years in the abortion debate. But, careful examination of the premise shows its flaws. What good is done to the person to be killed? In what way is the person better off? Who decides? If the patient is comatose or brain dead, how can we know whether *they* think they'll be better off?

Preserving and lengthening life is one thing—deciding when someone is better off without it is another. With medically dependent people, does the command, "Do unto others as you would have them do unto you," really amount to killing them? Or, are we obligated to befriend and comfort them?

The Killing That Nobody Does

That structure served to diffuse individual responsibility. In the entire sequence . . . there was at no point a sense of personal responsibility for, or even involvement in, the murder of another human being. Each participant could feel like no more than a small cog in a vast, officially sanctioned, medical machine.[1]
                                    —Robert Jay Lifton, M.D., speaking
                                          of the Nazi euthanasia project

In the German euthanasia project, which was killing handicapped, retarded, and other people before the "Final Solution" for the Jews began, not only was the killing thoroughly scientific and medicalized, it was also bureaucratic and incremental.

Medical ethics boards justified the killing. Legislators passed laws allowing it. Special review boards approved each case. Sometimes relatives requested euthanasia. Doctors reviewed medical records and listed a likely cause of death on the death certificates. Everyone was involved—but nobody did it.[2]

Today, we are asked to make deadly medical decisions under a cloud of misdirection. The medical associations, press, religious leaders, and opinion shapers all urge us to do the "compassionate" thing. No muss, no fuss, and no blood on our hands. We just sign a little DNR or organ donation form or request to stop extraordinary care—all of which are available because the legislature passed laws allowing it. A nurse will come in and add sedatives and anti-convulsants to the IV drip or a medical team will declare him brain dead and part out his organs in a dozen different directions so that others might live. A minister or social worker from the hospital will notify us when the end is near so we can be there for our friend's passing. The death certificate will reflect death from natural causes or from the particular disease from which he suffered. A dutiful obituary will appear in the paper. A pastor will read the eulogy and preside over the burial. Everyone will be involved—but no one actually kills him. It is all so medical, so scientific, so sanctified.

So long as no one is to blame, we do not have to accept responsibility—or do we? Culpability is not so easy to dodge. If we knew, or even should have known, that our actions were part of that chain of death, God knows it and we will face Him on it. Proverbs 24:11–12 tells us, "If thou forbear to deliver them that are drawn unto death, and those that are ready to be slain; If thou sayest, *Behold, we knew it not;* doth not he that pondereth the heart consider it? and he that keepeth thy soul, doth not he know it? and shall not he render to every man according to his works?" (emphasis added)

Religious Rites

They go to heaven anyway.
                —A Christian explaining why saving
                babies from abortion is unnecessary

Having been involved in the battle to end abortion, I have probably heard just about every excuse for inaction by Christians that is imaginable (and probably many you could not even imagine). But, the excuse that the babies go to heaven anyway has to be one of the most disturbing.

First of all, it is centered on a debatable doctrine. Not all Christians believe that statement is true. But, even if it were provably true, wouldn't it also mean that we should not try to help Christians who are being persecuted in Communist China or in Moslem countries. After all, if they are Christians who are being killed by the Communists or Moslems, they are just going to heaven anyway. This is pretty cold reasoning. It would also justify killing every new Christian just after he made an altar call. Save them the trouble of having to live in this old, corrupted world, right?

Of course, the argument is ludicrous. However, it finds revival in the euthanasia movement—especially when the target is a believer. Medical staff are often aware of the religious beliefs of both patient and family. Many can "speak the language," as it were, as part of their training in dealing with grieving families. They can offer a little "religious" assistance in making the decision to "pull the plug" if the patient is going to be with God. And, they may throw in a little something about "making their death meaningful" when they approach you to part out their organs—so he can "live on and help others." Ministers may be invited in to add to the religious aura and even offer special religious rites to help the grieving family. Already, one group of ministers in Portland, Oregon, has launched a healing ritual complete with lighting candles and "statements of affirmation" for women who have killed their own children through abortion.[3]

But the "healing" they offer is centered on the family, not the patient. Their "compassion" is reserved for those who are not afflicted by disease. Religious-sounding excuses for killing someone are insufficient. No amount of knowing that they'll be in heaven or that their organs will help others will justify the shedding of innocent blood. We, as Christians, have very specific obligations to other people. Those must be followed regardless of emotional responses or reasonings about tragic circumstances.

"Letting Go"

As mentioned previously, old Daniel, an aging alcoholic, was asked to sign a "do-not-resuscitate" order when he was taken to the nursing home after his second stroke. Officials told him he would not be admitted without that signature. Lisa, a friend, would not let him sign the form and insisted that a lawsuit would follow if he was refused a place in the institution. Another stroke soon made Daniel incapable of response. The medical staff claimed that he was not even aware of anything going on around him. Lisa didn't believe it.

At one point, Lisa called in a minister for Daniel's comfort. The minister, however, tried to make Lisa feel guilty by telling her that she was in denial and was not "letting go" of Daniel. Worse, he then went into Daniel's room and began telling him that allowing him to die was really the best thing for him. During the minister's little sales job for death, Daniel became so increasingly and obviously agitated that the nursing staff had to sedate him. In fact, he became similarly agitated every time someone talked about allowing him to die. Lisa asked, "If Daniel is not aware, why do you have to sedate him at times like this?"

This is a true story. Lisa was a friend of mine. And, she cared deeply for Daniel, though he had been a stranger not long before. But, the professionals wanted to make her feel guilty about caring. She was "in denial" about Daniel's impending death, they said. She was selfish for refusing to let go. Evidently, even Daniel, in his alleged nonresponsive state, was also in denial. Perhaps, he, too, was being selfish and refusing to let go.

But, Lisa was just trying to keep these people from killing Daniel. Apparently, Daniel, in his own way, seemed to show that he agreed with Lisa's attempts. This story perfectly illustrates one of the last refuges of the Thanaphile scoundrel—guilt. They will try to make you feel guilty for trying to save a life. Pastors are particularly useful to the deathmongers for this duty. It is they who can best warp the moral issues that compel you to save life into dirty, little, selfish egotistical exercises.

But, saving lives is the true moral imperative. Even if your motives are mixed, there is no shame in that. Of course, you want your mother, father, brother, friend, or neighbor alive! Nothing could be more natural. Would it be a biblical virtue to not care? Wanting people to live is a holy desire. It is a recognition of the *value* of that human being—whether you know them or not. Don't let the pious platitudes and penny-ante psychoanalysis of the Thanaphiles deter you from protecting the defenseless.

Nice Nazis

He was capable of being so kind to children, to have them become fond of him, to bring them sugar, to think of small details in their daily lives, and do things we would genuinely admire. . . . And then, next to that, . . . the crematoria smoke, and these children, tomorrow or in a half an hour, he is going to send them there. Well, that is where the anomaly lay.[4]

—Auschwitz prisoner-doctor describing Nazi doctor Josef Mengele

As some of the Nazi concentration camp survivors will tell you, there were even nice Nazis. Their victims were, nonetheless, dead. There were a multitude of reasons for their niceness. Some actually believed they were sending the Jews—as they helped load them on the trains—to a relocation center where they would have their own farms and businesses. Others just thought it was best for them not to know and suffer the anxiety as they got on the trains or headed for the gas chambers. Some Nazi doctors truly thought national socialism (nazism) and racial purification was a "world blessing" (Weltbegluckung) and that their social engineering was a good thing. Still others felt that using prisoners as guinea pigs was justified because the prisoners were going to die anyway or have terrible lives in the labor camp.

Mengele was nice to kids. He was civilized. Who knows why he behaved nicely at all? And who cares—once it becomes evident what he was *doing* while being nice.

The same is true of Thanaphiles today. Many are nice, well-meaning people, who will end up killing you or your friends in the name of doing a good thing. Many are genuinely convinced that what they are doing is best for society, or that it is best for you not to know about potentially life-saving procedures since you wouldn't have a good quality of life anyway.

Remember, the Thanaphiles will not be drooling, cackling demoniacs with wild eyes and sharpened teeth. They will be ordinary doctors or medical staff. Many will be very compassionate, caring, nice, understanding people. They will soothe you with all the practical and even spiritual reasons why killing your neighbor is a good thing. They won't approach you with the proposition to murder someone, but to "let go" of someone, to "allow them to die," to do what's best for them.

The devil appears as an angel of light (2 Cor. 11:14). How successful do you think the devil would be in tempting people if he came up and said, "Hey, why don't you rebel against God, commit adultery against your wife, and follow me to hell?" The same is true here. The proposition to kill your relative, friend, or neighbor will come in a reasoned, pseudoscientific, and compassionate cloak. Don't be taken unaware.

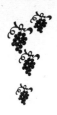

Chapter Thirteen

Closing the Bloodgates

If ideas have consequences, we need to have the right ideas. In the maze called medical ethics, the promoters of pagan ethics mask their ideas by deliberate sleight of tongue and by playing upon our emotions, our confusion over medical technology, and our lack of medical knowledge.

But, while technologies and terminology may be complex, right and wrong are not. What is needed is a means of slicing through the dark and swirling morass and finding the simple truths needed to make godly decisions.

In the Scriptures, there are both commands and principles. And, as the old saying goes, "Obey the commands and practice the principles." This is also true of most medical decisions involving life and death. There are usually one or two simple central commands or precepts from the Bible which contain the answer to your question—if you will perceive it through the confusing tangle of peripheral things that are thrown at you.

This means we have to diligently search for those principles in the Word of God. In this chapter, we will look at many of the most important scriptural considerations that may be involved in making these decisions. The list here will not be exhaustive because there may be future developments in medicine which hinge on other principles. But, I believe that if we diligently search (Matt. 7:7) and ask God's wisdom in prayer (James 1:5), we will be able to discern the right decision.

The hard part will be to implement that decision. There will be difficulties. Medical people will pressure you. Family members may resist. Even *you* will sometimes balk. After all, the decision may entail *great* sacrifices in time and money for you and your family. Or, it could mean continued pain for the patient. I don't want to either glamorize or be overly negative about this. Probably the majority of these life-affirming decisions will not create terrible conflicts or burdens—but some will. But, isn't this true in any area of obedience to God?

Obeying God

If ye love me, keep my commandments.
                                                        —John 14:15

The first of the two great commandments is to love God with our whole mind, soul, and might. As the quote above indicates, our love for God is proven by our obedience to Him. There are many things that can confuse our obedience to God, the most powerful of which are our emotions. Sometimes, forbidden acts feel right. In our society, adultery is often excused because of love, theft, because of injustice.

But, the Word of God is a firmer foundation than that. We, as believers, know that we, and our emotions, are corrupted by the fallen state of man. We therefore know that we cannot trust emotions as a guide. Yet, often this is the very thing we do.

Most of us don't have a problem with the commandment against committing adultery. We would not accept any excuses for such behavior. But, with today's medical ethics, we often find palatable excuses for killing. Compassion for the person who is in pain or dying tugs at our mind. Sorrow for the suffering of other family members enters the equation.

However, if we are to make godly decisions, we have to remember that obedience to God is the prime directive. Even what we might mistakenly call love for our neighbor—in following the second great commandment—cannot interfere, for those things we do in obedience to God will always be in accordance with true love for our neighbor. This is our first guide in making medical decisions for ourselves or others.

In His Image

And God said, Let us make man in our image, after our likeness: and let them have dominion over the fish of the sea, and over the fowl of the air, and over the cattle, and over all the earth, and over every creeping thing that creepeth upon the earth. So God created man in his own image, in the image of God created he him; male and female created he them.

—Genesis 1:26–27

God has made human beings in His image. This image encompasses body, soul, and spirit. Because of this we must treat human beings in a very special way. Since the beginning, Christians (not to mention the Jews) always chose respectful ways to dispose of their dead. The Romans, on the other hand, did so only for the wealthy and powerful. Slaves were tossed in the dump.

We should remember that God created people in His own image. The argument that we "put down" animals does not apply to humans, since animals are not made in the image of God. Animals do not have a moral sense. They cannot fornicate or steal because they have not been given moral bounds and a moral sense. Nor are people guilty of murder when they kill an animal for food. Though one might say the animal is innocent, it is not so because it cannot be guilty. This is precisely why we don't treat people as barnyard animals.

While living, people are not to be killed or injured for light or transient causes; however, there are times when these things are biblically justified. During legal and lawful punishment for crimes, the Bible allows severe punishment. But, God prohibits the shedding of innocent blood. Capital punishment, justifiable wars, self-defense, and defense of others are the biblical exceptions to the prohibition on killing. In such cases, the blood shed cannot be considered innocent. The unborn child, the comatose, or the brain dead person are judicially innocent. There is no lawful way before God to bring about, directly or indirectly, the end of their lives. The fact that they need assistance in breathing or eating by artificial means does not change that fact. If we are *able* to help, we should do it. And, once help has begun, we ought to continue it as long as we have the capability.

Innocent Blood

So shalt thou put away the guilt of innocent blood from among you, when thou shalt do that which is right in the sight of the LORD.
—Deuteronomy 21:9

The concept of innocent blood is central to how believers are to treat other people. While we know that all men have sinned and that none is innocent before God, the Scriptures prohibit the killing of those who have not been found *judicially* guilty. This is the foundation of the common law presumption of innocence as well as the American idea of due process of law. Our laws, originally reflecting the Judeo-Christian teachings, made us presume that a person was innocent until proven guilty.

No one is suggesting that this was scrupulously followed. Men, including those in authority, are still fallen creatures, but at least the principle and the ideal were sought after. In our subject, as I noted earlier, the medically dependent are judicially innocent. No one has the right before God to take their lives.

Your Neighbor

And the second [commandment] is like unto it, Thou shalt love thy neighbour as thyself.
—Matthew 22:39

This was the yardstick given by Jesus Christ. It wasn't how much we gave to missions, or how compassionate we were toward the starving in Somalia, or our emotional outbursts over the terrible things happening in Bosnia. It was how we treated the

people with whom we came into contact. The friend
or relative who is hospitalized is your neighbor.
There is no way to escape this fact.

Look at the parable of the Good Samaritan.
Jesus plainly tells us that the man who had fallen
prey to the robbers was the Samaritan's neighbor.

We can assume the victim was in pretty bad
shape. Maybe the Samaritan could have said, "He's
going to die anyway" and left him there, only noti-
fying the authorities at the end of his journey. Maybe
the victim could have been called brain dead, or the
Samaritan could have thought about the scarce
medical resources and the financial burden the victim would be. After all, when he had done all he
could for the man, it still was by no means certain
that the man would live at all or that he wouldn't
end up a cripple. Why leave money behind and
promise an uncertain amount of money in the future for this man's recovery? The Samaritan *loved*
his neighbor. The victim was of uncertain medical
prognosis. He was time-consuming. He was expensive—and promised to be more so. And, he was a
stranger. Does this tell us anything about our responsibilities?

The Afflicted, Oppressed, Needy, Fatherless, and Widows

*Open thy mouth, judge righteously, and plead the
cause of the poor and needy.*

—Proverbs 31:9

Not only are we to watch out for our neighbor,
but Scripture tells us to take particular care of the
afflicted, oppressed, and needy. These are people

who cannot pay you back. When Jesus was asked by John the Baptist's men if He was the One they sought, He listed off several proofs that He was the Christ: Healing the sick, cleansing the lepers, giving sight to the blind, and preaching the gospel to the poor. Did you ever wonder why that last one was a sign of Jesus being the Christ?

I suspect it was because of the audience He was preaching to. Many preached, but few targeted the poor with their message. The poor have no prospect of repaying you. How can a ministry survive unless it targets people who can be *supporters*, one might ask. Wouldn't you want to aim for people of influence so that the good news could trickle down as it became known that this or that famous person were a believer? That wasn't what Jesus did.

In like manner, we are to understand that not only the words of the gospel but the acts of mercy that God empowers us to do should be available to the meanest of men. Consider the current mania for only giving medical help to those who will continue to be productive in society. Isn't that the same as only helping those who can pay you back? Jesus said that even the pagans do that much (Matt. 5:46–47).

Take the time to carefully consider the terms listed above. The Scripture have a real focus on our responsibilities to these people. We are to heal the sick—not kill them. We are to comfort the afflicted—not allow them to die. We are to help the fatherless—not turn our backs and ignore that they are being killed. We are commanded to rescue those being dragged to death (Prov. 24:11–12), speak up for the defenseless (Prov. 31:9), comfort those who need it (1 Cor. 1:4), assist the fatherless and the widow (James 1:27). All of these apply very well to the medically dependent—especially those who have no friends or resources.

Closing the Bloodgates

Rescue those being led away to death; hold back those staggering toward slaughter.
—Proverbs 24:11

The task appears daunting. But, remember that God is not expecting you to change the entire medical system and alter the current course of medical ethics alone. He wants you to love your neighbor. If doing that helps to solve these larger problems, wonderful; if not, you have obeyed God. However, even knowing that you are to love one single, medically needy neighbor can be overwhelming. The medical opposition—even the religious opposition—may be great. Doctors and other medical staff may resist you or treat you with disdain. Pastors and other religious people may try to reason with you. You will have to stand your ground based upon the principles found in the Scriptures.

Consider Mike McHugh, a Vermont pastor and prolife leader. He became aware of the plight of Ronald Comeau, a thirty-year-old transient who had tried to hang himself in the holding cell in the Bennington City Police Department. The attempt had left him comatose—possibly a level eight on the Glasgow Scale. It wasn't long after a cursory attempt to locate the man's father that Comeau was appointed a guardian. The guardian pushed through the process to remove nutrition and hydration. McHugh appealed to the court, but was denied because he could not show "a direct interest" in Comeau's welfare. "The good Samaritan didn't know the guy in the ditch either," McHugh told the judge. "For them to tell a pastor he has no direct interest in the life of a guy who is being murdered is outrageous."

McHugh immediately appealed to the Vermont Supreme Court. The court ordered feeding to resume until a hearing could be held—in less than a week. McHugh and John Goyette, a fellow pastor, drove to Maine, found Comeau's father, and returned with him to Vermont just minutes before the hearing was to commence. Comeau's life was saved by the willing and persistent action of Christians who saw the transient stranger as a neighbor created in the image of God.[1] This is one example of how lives have been saved, but, to do likewise, you must be prepared.

In order to press your case, you will have to familiarize yourself with the medical issues you are facing. This may not be as hard as you think. There are many resources out there in layman's language that will tell you all about medical conditions. There are also resources like the *Physician's Desk Reference* (PDR) where you can find out many things you need to know about any drugs that might be used in your circumstance—or that of your relative, friend, or neighbor. Dr. Robert Mendelsohn says that reading even medically oriented materials is not all that difficult. "Anybody with an eighth grade education and a dictionary can read *any* medical book. Even doctors will testify that patients always seem to be able to pick out and understand the parts that they *must* know."[2]

In fact, as preparation for any future forays into the medical field, I recommend you read Dr. Mendelsohn's book as soon as you finish this one. Even knowledge, though, will not save your neighbor unless used properly. If someone is in the hospital, it is best if a friend is there monitoring his or her progress as close to around-the-clock as possible. Friends and family can also be recruited to keep close watch on the patients. Do not blindly accept the medical pronouncements of the medical staff. Naturally, the medical staff will try to tell you that you are disturbing the patient, despite the fact that you are just trying to protect the patient. Don't give up your ground. You may be the only person who stands between the relative and the "non-treatment" of the doctor's choice.

To Thy House

Is not this the fast that I have chosen? to loose the bands of wickedness, to undo the heavy burdens, and to let the oppressed go free, and that ye break every yoke? Is it not to deal thy bread to the hungry, and that thou bring the poor that are cast out to thy house? when thou seest the naked, that thou cover him; and that thou hide not thyself from thine own flesh?

—Isaiah 58:6–7

This verse has some scary words in it. Among the scariest is "to *thy* house." God is commending some very personal action on behalf of the needy. It would be so much easier if he said to send the poor to the Salvation Army, which you already support with your tax-deductible donations, instead of dealing *thy* bread to them and taking them to *thy* house.

For those we are trying to protect from death, it will be difficult to have them in any kind of institution where we can be absolutely assured that they will not be "selectively non-treated" to death. If you can find one, that's good. But, in the event you cannot, it may be necessary to take them into your own home. This might mean learning how to feed, bathe, give medications, and even keep various machines going for the person. In fact, most hospitals have training for lay people to do just those sorts of things. This is far cheaper than placing the person in any kind of institution. Of course, the expense may to some degree come out of you. You are personally responsible for a lot of work. It makes having an outside life more difficult. But, then, none of the "promises in the Book" we Christians are so fond of claiming says we'll have an outside life. I believe, however, we are told to pick up our cross and follow Him. And, think about it for a minute. Where would you prefer to be if you were incapacitated or dying? Among friends and relatives, or in a hospital? Do unto others . . .

Dealing with the Dying

Give strong drink unto him that is ready to perish . . .

—Proverbs 31:6a

Some years ago, when a suggestion arose at congressional hearings that heroin be legalized as a pain killer for the terminally ill, a congressman said that he was afraid the patients would become addicted. As ludicrous as that worry was, it was the reason cited and the drug was never approved for those purposes.

The Scripture, as cited above, recommends giving a dying person something to ease his pain. This is a fundamental issue in care for the dying. Remember, while these people may be *dying* they are not *dead*. What they most need, especially in the final stages is "comfort care."

"Comfort care" consists of warmth, appropriate food, water, being kept clean, medications (like antibiotics), and pain control. This care might also be used in caring for any nonresponsive (comatose or brain dead) person. While most people do not die in pain, and most who do die in minimal pain of the sort that can be controlled with aspirin, the science of pain control has advanced to the point where almost all pain can be made at least bearable with proper palliative care. Unfortunately, most doctors have not been trained in this. If it is to be had, it can be learned from people in the hospice movement (check your phone book). One of the complex questions the Thanaphiles are fond of raising in cases like this is about the fact that most painkilling medications will shorten life—especially when higher dosages are necessary.

There is some truth to this. A dying patient who is on a morphine drip may die several hours or days early due to the suppressive effect that morphine has on the respiratory system. When the breathing apparatus is deteriorating, this suppressive effect will cause the respiratory system to fail earlier. The option, of course, is to have the person in agony a few hours or days longer. The Thanaphiles would argue that giving them the morphine is tantamount to euthanasia and that they are just carrying that logic to its natural conclusion when there is the demand for euthanasia or physician-assisted suicide.

The comparison is false. First of all, the morphine drip was given in an attempt to control pain, not with the intent to kill. The slightly early death is an *unintended consequence* of a good we were trying to accomplish. We are only seeing to a dying person's comfort, not trying to kill them. Notice the difference between what the Thanaphiles recommend and what is indicated by comfort care. They say to starve the hungry and give no hydration to the thirsty. Comfort care does the opposite. The Scriptures say to *feed* the hungry and *give drink* to the thirsty. Which advice sounds more like God's Word?

Using the Sense God Gave You

Not all medical decisions are perfectly clear-cut in Scripture. This is where prayer and common sense come in. At times, you may have to do things that seem contrary to what you have learned in this book. For instance, there are times when you will not want to feed a patient. Some people who are close to death find food intolerable. It is more an irritant and a discomfort than a help—whether it comes from a spoon or a tube. In cases like this, we don't insist on food being given. Intravenous fluids and nutrients are probably enough so that starvation or dehydration are not occurring. However, remember that a person who cannot or will not drink fluids may need to have his mouth moistened for comfort's sake.

These are not really "gray areas." Don't let the Thanaphiles use them as leverage to get you to do something that would result in death for your friend. Remember, don't do anything (or fail to do anything) that you know will result in death or that is *intended* to cause death.

Don't Forget the Person

In all this wrangling with the medical people and working on ways to assist the patient, don't forget the person that is inside. This is especially easy to do with nonresponsive people. Our human natures tend to ignore people and things that don't respond to us after a while. But, it is essential for you to go to great lengths to treat these people as human. Hold birthday parties for them, talk to them, read to them, greet them first thing in the morning just like you would any other friend or neighbor.

Be aware that *they* may be aware. Do not allow others, including medical staff or friends, to talk about them as if they were not there. We have absolutely no idea what these people are capable of in their nonresponsive state. Love your neighbor as yourself!

Christians in Medicine

For unto whomsoever much is given, of him shall be much required: and to whom men have committed much, of him they will ask the more.

—Luke 12:48b

Until now, we have looked almost exclusively at the role of the average, nonmedical Christian in protecting himself and others from medically induced death. But, there is a whole class of people who have been overlooked—Christians in medicine.

When I look at this, quite frankly, I see little hope. Considering the dearth of response from this group to the holocaust of abortion as well as the lack of any visibility in the euthanasia debate, I don't see much help from these quarters. I once attended a rock-solid, conservative, evangelical church where one of the board members, a doctor, quite openly admitted doing abortions. In the Oregon election containing the physician-assisted suicide measure, the Catholic church was just about alone on the field opposing the measure. Christian medical groups were almost nowhere to be found.

Sadly, many Christians have come down on the same side of many of the issues as the Thanaphiles. They are so immersed in their knowledge of science that they have forgotten their knowledge of godly principle. But, if the average Christian is responsible to love his neighbor and to take care of those who are medically dependent, the Christian doctor or nurse has multiplied responsibilities before God. Their special knowledge and position makes them able to do more and, therefore, responsible to do more. The question for them is: What are you willing to do? Will you risk your job, or your prestige? I know of one doctor who lost his prestige and any influence he had at the hospital where he worked because he would not view patients as organ farms.

This Christian doctor was called by the relative of a girl in her late teens who had gotten in an accident and had been declared brain dead. The parents had already been approached for the organs, but they agreed to hold off until this doctor came. The parents, who were Christians, were overwrought because they felt their daughter was unsaved. But, they had been convinced by the medical staff that she would never recover and that at least the organ donations would make some sense of the tragic circumstances.

The doctor had no standing in the hospital where the girl lay, but would not be dissuaded. He gathered all the family and friends (about forty of them) into the tiny room, led the group in prayer, and began to preach the gospel to the girl. At the end, when he asked the girl if she would accept Christ, tears began to flow from her eyes. This convinced the parents that she was not dead so they decided not to allow her to be unplugged.

She died two weeks later, but in the interim, about a dozen of those who had been in the room during that fateful episode came to know Christ. The medical staff was saddened by the waste of good organs, but the angels in heaven were rejoicing over the soul which was saved.

The Christian doctor? Well, the word got around about what he had done, and he lost any prestige and influence he had built during his years in practice. He says it was worth it. So, the questions remain for the Christian doctors in America. Will you feed the hungry as the Word commands when the chart says "no nutrition and hydration"? Will you treat a person as dead who still has a pulse and blood pressure? How will you treat patients when they aren't pretty or useful or responsive? A Christian doctor may be able to run and hide in a specialty where such questions never arise, but is

that the extent of his duty? Will God accept that?
I think not.

Remember, caring for the sick was not always a
profession—it was originally a ministry. During the
Middle Ages, men and women dedicated their lives
to hospital orders to care for the sick and the dying.
It was not a matter of income, but a matter of
vocation.

What about Him?

*Then Peter, turning about, seeth the disciple whom
Jesus loved following; which also leaned on his breast at
supper, and said, Lord, which is he that betrayeth thee?*

*Peter seeing him saith to Jesus, Lord, and what
shall this man do?*

*Jesus saith unto him, If I will that he tarry till I
come, what is that to thee? follow thou me.*

—John 21:20–21

As I mentioned before, it is not likely that it
will be possible for you to change the course of
modern medical ethics. Your actions may, in sum,
help to do that. Your primary goal, however, is to
obey God in the circumstances that present themselves to you.

None of this depends upon the obedience of
others. Just like in the verses quoted above, their
obedience is not your concern. In the prolife battle,
I see a great absence of fellow Christians—Christians who should be doing *something* but are doing
nothing. While distressing to see, this has no bear-
ing on what I am to do. It would be wonderful if
Christian doctors, nurses, pastors, and laymen would
suddenly become active in putting feet to their faith

to save life—unborn or born. But, if it doesn't happen, the job still lies before me. Even if I can't change the culture, I can save a life.

Historically, the culture has been turned and changed by a very tiny minority of Christians willing to go against the flow—even the flow of the Church. And, those people often found their obedience very costly. Often, there was direct persecution. But, as the saying goes, "Pioneers get the arrows; settlers get the land." There is no other way to put it.

This is a battle that only God can win, and He will win it according to His plan.

Ora et labora [Pray and work].

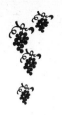

Notes

Chapter One

1. Barbara DeJong, *Tracing the Jewish Disporia* (Amsterdam: The English Press, 1967), cited in George Grant, *The Quick and the Dead* (Wheaton, IL: Crossway Books, 1991), 95.

Chapter Two

1. Tom Philip and Joanne Grant, "Brain-dead woman gives birth," *Oregonian* (31 July 1986).

2. Willard Gaylen, "Harvesting the Dead," *Harper's* (September 1974): 23.

3. A. Mohandas and S. Chou, "Brain Death: A Clinical and Pathological Study," *Journal of Neurosurgery* (1971): 211.

4. Nat Hentoff, "Should Paul Brophy Have Been Put to Death?" *Village Voice* (22 September 1987): 36.

5. Joseph Fletcher, "Indicators of Humanhood: A Tentative Profile of Man," *International Hastings Center Report* (November 1972): 1.

6. Oz Hopkins, "Team transplants first heart at OHSU," *Oregonian* (5 December 1985): A-1.

7. Paul Byrne and Paul M. Quay, *On Understanding Brain Death* (Omaha, NE: Nebraska Coalition for Life Educational Trust Fund, n.d.).

Chapter Three

1. "19 Arrested In Hospital Near Cruzan," *St. Louis Post-Dispatch* (19 December 1990). Paul deParrie, "Nancy Cruzan Killed In 'Legal' Action," *Advocate* (February 1991): 3.

2. Associated Press, "Mother, 24, no longer comatose," *Oregonian* (31 January 1989).

3. Callista Gould, "Comatose mother gives birth then awakens," *Life Advocate* (September 1991): 11.

4. *Merritt's Textbook of Neurology* (Eighth Edition), Lewis P. Rowland, ed. (Philadelphia, PA: Lea & Febiger, 1989), 373.

Chapter Four

1. Roy Hoopes, "When it's time to leave: Can society set an age limit for health care?" *Modern Maturity* (August–September 1988): 38.

2. Donald Robinson, "The Crisis In Our Nursing Homes," *Parade Magazine* (16 August 1987): 12.

3. Fred Bayles and Scott McCartney, "Guardians of the elderly," *Oregonian* (20 September 1987): A2.

4. Wolf Wolfensberger, Ph.D., "The Extermination of Handicapped People in World War II Germany," *Ethical Issues Revisited* (n.d.).

5. *TIPS*, Division of Special Education and Training, Syracuse University, New York (April 1988), 11.

6. Christine Gorman, "The Doctor's Crystal Ball," *Time* (10 April 1995): 60.

7. "Dutch televise 'immoral' game show," *Life Advocate* (February 1994): 8.

8. David Stewart, Ph.D., "Amniocentesis: Search and Destroy," *Life Advocate* (March 1993): 44.

9. Robert Lee Hotz, "New Strides, Hard Choices in Genetics," *Atlanta Journal and Constitution* (25 January 1988): 5.

10. Philip Reilly, *The Surgical Solution: A History of Involuntary Sterilization in the United States* (Johns Hopkins University Press, 1991).

Chapter Five

1. From a list of the effects of starvation and dehydration provided to trial judge David Kopelman in a "death with dignity" case. Reported by Nat Hentoff, "Come Sweet Death," *Village Voice* (29 September 1987): 36.

2. Joseph P. Shapiro, "Others saw a victim, but Ed Roberts didn't," *U.S. News & World Report* (27 March 1995): 7.

3. Christopher Martinez, "Was it All Right to Starve Marjorie Nighbert?" *Our Sunday Visitor* (23 April 1995): 3.

4. Patrick O'Neill, "The Complex Case of Baby Ryan," *Oregonian* (19 February 1995): D-1. Paul deParrie, "Interstate flight . . . to save a life!" *Life Advocate* (February 1995): 12.

5. "Parents of 'Infant Doe' find no peace of mind," *Chicago Tribune* (18 April 1983), Section 1, p. 3.

6. Daniel Callahan, *The Hastings Center Report* (October 1983) quoted in Nat Hentoff, "Rx: No Food/No Water," *Village Voice* (6 October 1987): 33.

Chapter Six

1. Nigel Davies, *Human Sacrifice in History and Today* (New York: William Morrow, 1981), 25.

2. Garry Hogg, *Cannibalism and Human Sacrifice* (New York: Citadel Press, 1966).

3. Paul deParrie and Mary Pride, *Unholy Sacrifices of the New Age* (Wheaton, IL: Crossway Books, 1988), 15.

4. Davies, *Human Sacrifice,* 97.

5. Audrey K. Gordon, "Reaction to Gibson," *Mental Retardation* (August 1984).

6. Kathleen Stein, "Last Rites," *Omni* (September 1987): 59.

7. Eric Lichtblau, "Family Sues Over Use of Heart in Transplant," *Los Angeles Times* (21 April 1989).

8. Willard Gaylin, "Harvesting the Dead," *Harper's* (September 1974): 23.

9. "Court may redefine incompetent patients as 'dead,'" *Life Advocate* (November 1992): 22.

10. Ellen Goodman, "'Harvesting' for Organs Goes Too Far," *Oregonian* (11 December 1987).

11. Arthur Schafer, "Case of Infant Organ Donor Poses Dilemma," *Oregonian* (29 October 1987): E-2.

12. Arthur Schafer, "'Brain absent' babies pose transplant dilemma," *Toronto Globe and Mail* (16 July 1987).

13. Stein, "Last Rites."

14. Gwynne Dyer, "Charting the ethics of human spare parts," *Oregonian* (25 August 1988).

15. "India's Kidney Transplant Racket?" *Lancet* (11 February 1995): 376.

16. Shuen Zhi, Luk Yee, Fu Si-hon, and Vittoria D'Alessio, "Embryonic food of life," *Eastern Express* (12 April 1995).

17. Denise Hamilton, "She's having a baby to save her daughter's life," *Oregonian* (17 February 1990).

18. *Encyclopedia of Religion and Ethics*, vol. 3 (New York: Scribner's and Sons, 1911), 199.

Chapter Seven

1. Gerald Parshall, "Freeing the Survivors," *U.S. News & World Report* (3 April 1995): 51.

2. "Man in coma dies after medical experiment," *Oregonian* (29 February 1988).

3. Thomas H. Maugh II, "Transplants of Cells Aided Diabetics, Doctors Say," *Los Angeles Times* (12 April 1995).

4. Jenny Westberg, "D&X: Grim technology for abortion's older victims," *Life Advocate* (February 1993): 4.

5. Thomas Levenson, "The Heart of the Matter," *Discover* (February 1985): 82–87.

6. Suzanne Rini, *Beyond Abortion: A Chronicle of Fetal Experimentation* (Rockford, IL: Tan Books and Publishers, 1988), 1.

7. Rini, *Beyond Abortion*, 21.

8. Ibid.

9. Ibid.

10. Houston, Texas, Pro-Life Telephone Newsline (now defunct).

11. David Stewart, Ph.D., "Amniocentesis: Search and Destroy," *Life Advocate* (March 1993): 44.

12. Rini, *Beyond Abortion*, 3, 57, 147.

13. Rini, *Beyond Abortion*, 4.

14. Ibid., 3.

15. Shuen Zhi, Luk Yee, Fu Si-hon, and Vittoria D'Alessio, "Embryonic food of life," *Eastern Express* (12 April 1995).

16. Dan Medynaki, "A Conversation with Dr. Mike McCune: The Man Who Built a Better Mouse," *Bay Area Reporter* (6 April 1995): 20.

Chapter Eight

1. Robert Jay Lifton, M.D., *The Nazi Doctors: Medical Killing and the Psychology of Genocide* (San Francisco, CA: Basic Books, 1986), 71.

2. "Court To Say Who Decides On Unplugging Life Support," *Life Advocate* (July 1991): 10.

3. Paul A. Byrne, M.D., "Before you sign . . . on the dotted line," *Life Matters* (Winter 1992): 24–32.

4. CURE, 812 Stephen St., Berkeley Springs, WV 25411.

5. Earl Appleby, "DaNgeR—DNR!!!" *Life Matters* (Winter 1992): 12.

6. Ibid., 12–15.

Chapter Nine

1. Written by Dan Zimmerman, 1986.

2. From a 21 January 1992 open letter from Randall Terry, founder of Operation Rescue, quoting from a book by J.S. Conway, *The Nazi Persecution of the Churches, 1933–45* (n.p., n.d.).

3. Cathy Ramey, "Theologies In Conflict: The German Church and Dietrich Bonhoeffer," *Life Advocate* (April 1995): 10.

4. Luke 12:43.

5. David M. Kennedy, *Birth Control In America* (New Haven, CT: Yale University Press, 1971), 141.

6. Wolf Wolfensberger, Ph.D., "The Extermination of Handicapped People in World War II Germany," *Ethical Issues Revisited* (n.d.).

Chapter Ten

1. John 14:15; Matthew 7:20.

2. Nigel Davies, *Human Sacrifice in History and Today* (New York: William Morrow, 1981), 289–90.

3. Peter Singer, "Sanctity of Life or Quality of Life?" *Pediatrics* (July 1983): 128–29.

4. "Animal rights activist enters guilty pleas in arson, theft," *The Oregonian* (7 March 1995).

5. "A New Ethic for Medicine and Society," *California Medicine, The Western Journal of Medicine* (September 1970): 67.

Chapter Eleven

1. Albert Hoch & Karl Binding, *Permitting the Destruction of Unworthy Life* (Leipzig, Germany: n.p., 1922).

2. Nigel Davies, *Human Sacrifice in History and Today* (New York: William Morrow, 1981), 97.

3. Henry M. Morris, *The Long War Against God* (Grand Rapids, MI: Baker Book House, 1989).

4. Dr. Robert Mendelsohn, *Confessions of a Medical Heretic* (New York: Warner Books, 1979), 201.

5. Robert Jay Lifton, M.D., *The Nazi Doctors: Medical Killing and the Psychology of Genocide* (San Francisco, CA: Basic Books, 1986), xii.

6. Ibid., 18.

7. Ibid., 70.

8. Allan Parachini, "To kill a suffering patient," *Columbian* (19 July 1987).

9. Lifton, *The Nazi Doctors,* 258.

10. Maharishi Mahesh Yogi, *Inauguration of the Dawn of the age of Enlightenment* (Fairfield, IA: Maharishi International University Press, 1975), 47.

11. Hoch & Binding, *Permitting the Destruction.*

Chapter Twelve

1. Robert Jay Lifton, M.D., *The Nazi Doctors: Medical Killing and the Psychology of Genocide* (San Francisco, CA: Basic Books, 1986), 55.

2. Ibid.

3. "Women 'pastors' launch post-abortion 'healing' rituals," *Life Advocate* (April 1994): 24.

4. Lifton, *The Nazi Doctors,* 337.

Chapter Thirteen

1. Cathy Ramey, "Ronald Comeau: Dying for a Drink," *Life Advocate* (March 1994): 12. Sally Johnson, "Drifter's hospital case spurs euthanasia battle," *Washington Times* (10 March 1994): A-11.

2. Robert Mendelsohn, M.D., *Confessions of a Medical Heretic* (Chicago, IL: Contemporary Books, 1979), 40.

*We welcome comments from our readers.
Feel free to write to us at the following
address:*

Editorial Department
Huntington House Publishers
P.O. Box 53788
Lafayette, LA 70505

More Good Books from
Huntington House . . .

The Gender Agenda:
Redefining Equality
by Dale O'Leary

All women have the right to choose motherhood as their primary vocation. Unfortunately, the radical feminists' movement poses a threat to this right—the right of women to be women. In *The Gender Agenda*, author Dale O'Leary takes a spirited look at the feminist movement, its influence on legislation, and its subsequent threat to the ideals of family, marriage, and motherhood. By shedding light on the destructiveness of the radical feminists' world view, O'Leary exposes the true agenda of the feminist movement.

ISBN 1-56384-122-3

The First Lady:
A Comprehensive View of
Hillary Rodham Clinton
by Peter & Timothy Flaherty

Is Hillary Rodham Clinton a modern career woman or an out-of-control feminist? In this compelling account of her life, the authors suggest that Mrs. Clinton has been misrepresented in the media and misunderstood by both conservatives and liberals alike.

ISBN 1-56384-119-3

How to Be a Great Husband
by Tobias Jungreis

In marriage, failure is *not* an option. This user-friendly, upbeat guidebook gives men easy, practical suggestions on how to keep their marriages vibrant for a lifetime. Unique features include insightful lists of do's and don'ts and dozens of ideas drawn from a myriad of real-life situations. *How to Be a Great Husband* offers a refreshing approach to the "work" that is marriage, giving husbands invaluable insight on how to achieve success in this most important area of their lives—insight they can apply at the dinner table tonight! Read this book and discover how easy it is to be a "ten" among men.

ISBN 1-56384-120-7

Handouts and Pickpockets: Our Government Gone Berserk
by William P. Hoar

In his new book, William P. Hoar, a noted political analyst, echoes the sentiments of millions of Americans who are tired of being victimized by their own government. Hoar documents attacks on tradition in areas as diverse as the family and the military and exposes wasteful and oppressive tax programs. This chronicle of our government's pitiful decline into an overgrown Nanny State is shocking, but more shocking is Hoar's finding that this degeneration was no accident.

ISBN 1-56384-102-9

Legacy Builders:
Dad, What Does Your Life
Say to Your Wife and Children?
by Jim Burton

Today, feminism and changing economics make it difficult for men to understand their role in a society that seems to devalue their inherent qualities. Discover how men can build a legacy—and why America so desperately needs men to understand their role in the family and society.

ISBN 1-56384-117-7

ADD:
. . . the facts . . . the fables
. . . hope for your family
by Theresa Lamson

ADD (Attention Deficit Disorder) is often ridiculed by those cynics who deny its existence and by those who dogmatically insist that "spanking your child more" would correct all of his behavior problems. However, if you're the parent of a child who suffers this disorder, you are painfully aware that ADD is real. Cheer up! You're not a bad parent. You need hope, encouragement, and biblical solutions—this book offers you all three. In addition, the author shares valuable knowledge from the secular pool of current information.

ISBN 1-56384-121-5

Beyond Political Correctness: Are There Limits to This Lunacy?

by David Thibodaux, Ph.D.

Author of the best-selling *Political Correctness: The Cloning of the American Mind,* Dr. David Thibodaux now presents his long awaited sequel—*Beyond Political Correctness: Are There Limits to This Lunacy?* The politically correct movement has now moved beyond college campuses. The movement has succeeded in turning the educational system of this country into a system of indoctrination. Its effect on education was predictable: steadily declining scores on every conceivable test which measures student performance and increasing numbers of college freshmen who know a great deal about condoms, homosexuality, and abortion, but whose basic skills in language, math, and science are alarmingly deficient.

ISBN 1-56384-066-9

From Earthquakes to Global Unity: The End Times Have Begun

by Paul McGuire

From the controversial GATT treaty to the move toward a cashless society, we are witnessing events that have the capacity to alter our world significantly—and irrevocably. McGuire's fascinating research reveals how some of these changes might soon affect us all.

ISBN 1-56384-107-X

Combat Ready
How to Fight the Culture War
by Lynn Stanley

The culture war between traditional values and secular humanism is escalating. At stake are our children. The schools, the liberal media, and even the government, through Outcome-Based Education, are indoctrinating our children with moral relativism, instead of moral principles. *Combat Ready* offers sound advice about how parents can protect their children and restore our culture to its biblical foundation.

ISBN 1-56384-074-X

Out of Control—
Who's Watching Our Child
Protection Agencies?
by Brenda Scott

This book of horror stories is true. The deplorable and unauthorized might of Child Protection Services is capable of reaching into and destroying any home in America. No matter how innocent and happy your family may be, you are one accusation away from disaster. Social workers are allowed to violate constitutional rights and often become judge, jury, and executioner. Every year, it is estimated that over 1 million people are falsely accused of child abuse in this country. You could be next, says author and speaker Brenda Scott.

ISBN 1-56384-080-4

Freud's War with God:
Psychoanalysis vs. Religion
by Dr. Jack Wright, Jr.

Freud's hostility to religion was an obsession: he dismissed all religious belief as a form of mental illness—a universal neurosis—and devoted his life's work to attacking it in whatever form it might appear. No other single theorist has had the impact on psychiatrists, psychologists, and social workers as has Sigmund Freud. Dr. Jack Wright demonstrates how his influence can be felt in such varied phenomena as gay rights, outcome-based education, and the false memory syndrome—all elements of the culture war that rebel against God and religious orthodoxy.

ISBN 1-56384-067-7

The Media Hates Conservatives:
How It Controls the Flow of Information
by Dale A. Berryhill

Here is clear and powerful evidence that the liberal-leaning news media brazenly attempted to influence the outcome of the election between President George Bush and Candidate Bill Clinton. Through a careful analysis of television and newspaper coverage, this book confirms a consistent pattern of liberal bias (even to the point of assisting the Clinton campaign). The major media outlets have taken sides in the culture war. Through bias, distortion, and the violation of professional standards, they have opposed the traditional values embraced by conservatives and most Americans—to the detriment of our country.

ISBN 1-56384-060-X

Health Begins in Him:
Biblical Steps to Optimal Health and Nutrition
by Terry Dorian, Ph.D.

This book is offered as a resource for all those seeking knowledge about how to change their lives in ways that will enable them to preserve and maintain optimal health. Health and nutrition aficionados will also find this volume essential, thanks to the guidelines, scientific studies, and testimonials. Clear, concise, and lively dialogue makes this a very readable directory on foods, food preparation, lifestyle changes, and suggestions for renewal. Terry Dorian, Ph.D. has been a whole-foods advocate for more than twenty years and conducts seminars that teach degenerative disease prevention and cures.

ISBN 1-56384-081-2

In His Majesty's Service:
Christians in Politics
by Robert A. Peterson

In His Majesty's Service is more than a book about politics. It's a look at how real men have worked out their Christian beliefs in the rough-and-tumble world of high-level government, war, and nation-building. From these fascinating portraits of great Western leaders of the past, we can discover how to deal with some of the most pressing problems we face today. This exciting, but historically accurate, volume is as entertaining as it is enlightening.

ISBN 1-56384-100-2

The Truth about
False Memory Syndrome

by James G. Friesen, Ph.D.

With his new book on false memory syndrome, Dr. Jim Friesen cuts through all the misinformation being bandied about on this subject. Through harrowing, yet fascinating, case studies—dealing with everything from sexual to Satanic ritual abuse—Friesen educates the reader on the most complex coping mechanism of the human psyche. A pioneer in the treatment of multiple personality disorder, Friesen dispels the myths surrounding FMS and victims of abuse as no tabloid or talk show can.

ISBN 1-56384-111-8

Outcome-Based Education:
The State's Assault
on Our Children's Values

by Peg Luksik & Pamela Hobbs Hoffecker

From the enforcement of tolerance to the eradication of moral absolutes, Goals 2000 enjoins a vast array of bureaucratic entities under the seemly innocuous umbrella of education. Unfortunately, traditional education is nowhere to be found in this controversial, strings-attached program. In this articulate and thoroughly documented work, Luksik and Hoffecker reveal the tactics of those in the modern educational system who are attempting to police the thoughts of our children.

ISBN 1-56384-025-1

The Blame Game:
Why Society Persecutes Christians
by Lynn Stanley

The liberal media is increasing its efforts to suppress Christian values and religious freedom. At the same time, liberal courts and organizations such as the NEA are working to eliminate religion from American culture. In *The Blame Game,* Lynn Stanley exposes the groups attacking the constitutional rights of Americans to tradition and freedom of religion. Also, she explains what these factions fear from mainstream America and why they seek to destroy it through their un-American system of wretched moral relativism.

ISBN 1-56384-090-1

Global Bondage:
The U.N. Plan to Rule the World
by Cliff Kincaid

The U.N. is now openly laying plans for a World Government—to go along with its already functioning World Army. These plans include global taxation and an International Criminal Court that could prosecute American citizens. In *Global Bondage,* journalist Cliff Kincaid blows the lid off the United Nations. He warns that the move toward global government is gaining ground and that it will succeed if steps are not taken to stop it.

ISBN 1-56384-103-7 Tradepaper
ISBN 1-56384-109-6 Hardcover